V

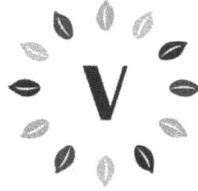

21stCentury Vegetarians.com

7 DAY VEGETARIAN STARTER KIT

Quick, Easy, Delicious Vegan Meals

Martha and Kamaal Theus

7 DAY VEGETARIAN STARTER KIT: Quick, Easy, Delicious Vegan Meals

Publisher:
21st Century Vegetarians
8939 S. Sepulveda Blvd, Suite 110-1024
Los Angeles, CA 90045
U.S.A.
www.21stcenturyvegetarians.com

Printed in the United States by CreateSpace a DBA of On-Demand Publishing, LLC

Cover design by Kamaal Theus, © 2010
Back cover author photo by Brennen Scott, www.brennenscott.com.

Library of Congress Control Number 2010937483

ISBN – 13: (Paperback) 978-0-9798688-1-8
ISBN – 10: (Paperback) 0-9798688-1-5

ISBN – 13: (eBook) 978-0-9798688-2-5
ISBN – 10: (eBook) 0-9798688-2-3

Disclaimer:
This book has been written based upon the personal experiences and information compiled by the authors. It was designed to provide information only and it is sold with the understanding that the publisher and the author are not engaged in rendering nutritional counseling or medical advice. If such advice is warranted, a competent professional should be consulted.

As is the nature with all consumer products, many new ones are introduced to the market while others are discontinued or their composition changed. Every effort has been made to ensure that the products recommended in this book are not only available but also suitable for vegetarians and vegans. However; due to the fact that we have no control over their formulas, you are urged to always read the labels and check the nutritional content to ensure that the products are still suitable for your lifestyle.

The registered trademarks displayed in this book are the sole property of their respective owners.

Also from Martha and Kamaal Theus

THROWIN' DOWN VEGETARIAN STYLE!

(Second Edition Coming Soon!)

Throwin' Down Vegetarian Style! is a vegetarian soul food cookbook and is the answer for those interested in changing their lives by changing their diets. It includes over 75 recipes, vegetarian product shopping guides, and the answers to common questions including "Where do you get your protein?", and "What do you eat?" The best part is that most of the recipes have more protein than average meat dishes, yet take less than 30 minutes to prepare! This is a great book for vegetarians AND non-vegetarians and is a perfect start for those thinking of transitioning to a vegetarian diet or to simply incorporate more healthy options in their lives for themselves and their families.

Mother/Daughter team Martha and Kamaal have "cracked the code" and taken the mystery and confusion out of vegetarian living by providing tips and recipes that are not only healthy but also very hearty and tasty and reminiscent of the foods we all grew up with. They have bridged the gap between eating "good" and eating "right." They don't believe you should have to choose between the two!

PRAISE FOR THROWIN' DOWN VEGETARIAN STYLE!

First of all, Martha had this book shipped out to me super fast. I have not been able to put it down since I received it. I am really enjoying her personal "down to earth" writing style so much! This cookbook is packed with great research information on the effects of diet on our health. The section on the health of African Americans is especially relevant.

The photos of her family and the food are just beautiful. I have already made her famous BBQ Fried Chickettes and my husband, myself, and our 2 year old son loved them. And my husband isn't even a vegetarian. I can't wait to try the rest of the recipes in this amazing collection. BUY THIS BOOK! **Valerie S. McGowan, California**

Awaken! This is a spiritual masterpiece for the mind, body, and soul. Not only are these food choices superior, but also tasty, delicious, appetizing, and pleasing to the eye. **Patrick Denson McGee, Los Angeles**

WOW!!!! Martha's vegetarian meals are so delicious. They are so tasty that one would not believe he is eating a vegetarian dish. GO AHEAD!!!! Try the recipes from this book and you will be HOOKED!!!! **Pat M. Gadsden, Alabama**

I have one word. WOW! Once I started reading I could not put it down. You completed a tremendous amount of research. Even with the extensive amount of research that you put in I love how you have also personalized your journey and decisions through personal and family experiences. I have already tried the Aztec recipe with the black beans and "chicken" and the barbecued chic-ketts. It is sooooooooo good! Oh.....another thing.....I really like when you make suggestions at the end or your recipes of what would be good to go with that particular meal. **Penny E., Baltimore, MD**

Yes, sometimes unusual things happen after a switch to a vegetarian diet. I've seen a number of cases in which the poor people broke out in violent attacks of good health, followed by bouts of physical exercise and sweet thoughts.

-Anonymous

Contents

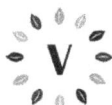

To become a vegetarian is to step into the stream which leads to nirvana.

-Buddha

1

Introduction

So many people I've met over the years are curious about our family and wonder how we've been able to maintain a vegetarian lifestyle for so long. On a daily basis, we get questions such as *"Where Do You Get Your Protein?"* (that's the #1 question!), *"How Long Have You Been Vegetarian?"*, *"What Do You Eat?"*, and even – *"But Don't You Still Eat Chicken?"*, to which I respond *"What plant does chicken come from?"* So, before we get into the details of how to use this 7 Day Vegetarian Starter Kit, I thought I would take a little time to tell you about our family and about our vegetarian approach.

Let's start with me – I am a native of Detroit, MI, graduated from the University of Michigan (Ann Arbor) with a degree in Accounting, and have lived in Los Angeles since 1983. People often ask me, *"Were you a vegetarian growing up?"* The answer is NO. My Mom is from the south and, to be honest, before I moved to California, I had only met one vegetarian - my boss at my first job scooping ice cream (making $1.65 an hour!) at the Northland Shopping Center in Detroit. She was Indian, and she and her entire family were vegetarian and practiced the Jain religion. I never asked her why they were vegetarian, and from my perspective, as a teenager in Detroit, being a vegetarian was a concept just as foreign to me as the land she came from *(I have since visited India several times so I no longer consider it a foreign land!)*.

After graduating college and moving to Los Angeles in 1983, I began my career as a Certified Public Accountant. One day (February 14, 1985 to be exact) my life changed so profoundly and took a course I never imagined in my wildest dreams. That was the day I met my (future) husband, Londale Theus. We met through my mother, who was working at the University of Southern California in cancer research. Londale was a campus Police Officer and often walked my mother to her car after she spent long hours in the lab. On this particular evening, I carpooled with my mother and when we got home late that night, she "endured" my lamenting about how on this particular Valentine's Day, I didn't have a date, much less flowers or a card from any of the 5 million or so potential suitors in Los Angeles. Not one....not even a phone call.....

She let me go on for some time before handing me a card from Londale. I remember thinking that it was pretty lame to get your only Valentine's Day card from your Mom! I was shocked to see that it was actually from Londale, and he wrote a short note along with his phone number. I called him the next day and we had a five hour conversation that changed my life forever.

He explained first and foremost what he was about and what he believed. The most amazing part, in my opinion, was that he was a vegetarian, and that it was a commitment he made in accordance with a spiritual path he was following. This took me by complete surprise, because as I mentioned, I had only met one vegetarian in my life and she most certainly was not a young Black man from South Central Los Angeles. For the first time, I met someone who "looked like me" but was a vegetarian. If nothing else, that intrigued me and I had to know more. I really cannot describe what happened, but by the end of that five hour conversation, I knew everything would be different. I felt as though some sort of veil had been lifted and I did not look at myself, the world, or its inhabitants in the same way. For the first time, I saw animals as living creatures with consciousness that were not put upon this planet simply to satisfy our appetites.

Londale and I met several times over the next few weeks and I grilled him about this philosophy and about all aspects of vegetarianism. On April 9, 1985, over 25 years ago, I ate my last animal at breakfast. It was a pig - or should I say part of a pig - pork chops to be exact! I used to eat meat three times a day and had NO PROBLEM eating leftover fried pork chops for BREAKFAST – can you imagine that? Well, on that day I don't know what shifted in my soul between breakfast and lunch, but something did and I have not eaten poultry, fish, eggs, or any type of meat since that morning in 1985. There was simply no turning back and there is no other way for me to live other than as a vegetarian for the rest of my life *(so don't let anyone tell you that it's impossible to convert to a vegetarian in one day – I am living proof that it is!)*

Things moved REALLY quickly after that! Londale and I were married on September 14, 1985 in Venice, California, just steps from the beach. Three days later, Kamaal (my daughter and co-author) was on her way to spoil our fun! Can you imagine getting married and pregnant within the same week? I was adjusting to my new husband, my new surroundings, my new in-laws, my new spiritual philosophy, my new diet, and my new baby growing inside of me. All of this at the tender age of twenty - two. It was a lot to deal with, to say the least!

All throughout my pregnancy I maintained a strict vegetarian diet. Nearly everyone around me told me that it was not safe, and that my baby would not be healthy if I didn't eat meat (in many ways 1985 was still the dark ages). Even though Londale was living proof that you could be healthy and strong as a vegetarian (he was a police officer and even won "The Toughest Cop Alive" competition which is a decathlon for police officers in California Police Olympics) he and I always heard the remark – *"But you guys weren't born vegetarian. Babies need meat and dairy in order to develop properly."* I would be lying to you if I said that this did not bother me and even scare me in some way. But I KNEW that my choice was a choice for compassion and that by choosing to honor the spirit in all of God's creatures, that He would reward me and my new baby with good health. My doctor (ironically a young University of Michigan grad – Go Blue!) supported my decision which was a great comfort to me as well.

Kamaal was born June 6, 1986. Five months later, Londale Jr. was on his way (I know - enough with the barefoot and pregnant jokes!) and was born on August 25, 1987. Bottom line, between September 1985 and August 1987 I was pregnant for 18 of those 23 months and did not compromise my vegetarian diet in any way. Both of my children were completely healthy at birth and are still healthy today, after 24 and 23 years respectively of being vegetarian by THEIR CHOICE. Londale Jr. is 6'6", weighs 200 pounds, played Division 1 college basketball, is now an actor and comedian, and has never eaten meat. Kamaal, while in college, played water polo and rugby, lived abroad in Costa Rica her freshman year and has never eaten meat. We never forced our way of life on them - we just demanded that they respect our choice and not bring meat of any kind into our home, just like alcohol and drugs were forbidden. We never fed them animals either - if we consider something poison for us, why would we feed it to our kids? Even still, we as parents always gave them the right to choose when they became older - we believe in being living examples and not making undue restrictions on our kids. This is a personal choice and we understand that they have to choose their own path. The fact that they are still vegetarian today is a testament to them and their understanding of why we believe what we believe.

Out of curiosity one day, I asked them when they were teenagers if they ever thought about at least trying meat since they had never had it and they had always heard *"you don't know what you're missing."* They both looked at me like I was crazy. They told me it was disgusting and cruel, and why would they want to eat dead animals now, after all these years? Obviously, being a vegetarian did not hurt their physical development at all so why eat meat now? Just recently, I was talking to my son about it (it seems that as a young actor and athlete, he is always explaining his diet) and he said, *"Mom....think about it.....name one disadvantage to a vegetarian diet....just one"*, and to be honest, I couldn't. That statement made it so simple - I believe my family is living proof that there are no disadvantages to the vegetarian lifestyle.

Kamaal's Perspective

For me, it was never a choice. Being a vegetarian is who I am, just like being a woman. I never thought of it as a choice but more as a part of my core being. Over the years, people have looked at me in bewilderment when I say, "I have never eaten meat." They are astonished by the fact that I "do not miss meat" or "never wanted to try it." How can I miss something that I have never tried? Why would I want to try something that I am not even remotely curious about?

The reality is that I am extremely happy and grateful for this way of life my parents have introduced me to. I could not think of living any other way. I could not think of a life more joyous than the one I am living right now; and vegetarianism is a key component to that joy, the foundation of it.

Our Approach

First and foremost, if you haven't figured this out already, THIS BOOK IS NOT JUST FOR VEGETARIANS. In fact, our approach works very well for those who are not vegetarian at all, but who are interested in knowing how to incorporate vegetarian options from time to time to add more variety or because they understand the overall benefits of the diet. This book and our two others *Throwin' Down Vegetarian Style (Second Edition)*, and *Meatless Mondays: 52 Weeks of Meat-Free Meals* provide a simple, easy to adopt approach that anyone can implement right away. And when I say *anyone*, I mean *anyone*. When I became a vegetarian over 25 years ago, I could not even boil water and could not imagine a meal without meat. Basically, I had spent all of my teenage and early adult years applying myself in school and work and as a result I never learned to cook – I just ate what my mother prepared, or when I left home (at age 17) and was suddenly on my own, I ate a lot of fast food and baloney sandwiches. After becoming vegetarian and getting married, and most importantly getting pregnant, I *had* to learn to cook in a manner that was in accordance with our beliefs, satisfied the cravings of my southern roots, and was fast and simple since I was a new wife, new mom, and had a new full-time job in public accounting.

Sound impossible? Not at all. Over the past 25 years I feel Kamaal and I have "cracked the code" and taken the mystery and confusion out of vegetarian living. Our books are full of easy to prepare, "down home" style recipes from common vegetarian items that can be found in most grocery stores. However, our approach, according to most vegetarian chefs, may be considered "cheating." What I mean by "cheating" is that I will use a ready-made vegetarian substitute in a heartbeat. I have absolutely no problem with the "mock meats" that are on the market today and do not feel as though I am "cheating" by using ready-made products that may resemble the "real thing." And it's not that I secretly crave meat. I don't. I have not eaten a dead animal or any part thereof in over 25 years and trust me, I don't miss it! But I would be lying if I said that I never liked the taste of certain foods, like (surprise!) fried chicken. So what did I do? I found what I consider to be the best chicken substitute on the planet (Gardein®), dipped it in batter, rolled it in flour, fried it up, dipped it in barbeque sauce, and voila! Barbeque Fried Chick'n was born! They are completely vegan (no animal products at all), free of cholesterol (cholesterol only comes from animal sources), and delicious. My husband loves them, my kids and their friends love them, and my meat eating friends literally dream about them (no joke)! And the best part is that most of these products have more protein than their meat "counterparts" (see *"Where Do You Get Your Protein"* in *Chapter Three: Vegetarian Myths – The Truth Revealed!*) for more information. So what if it tastes like the "real thing?" In my opinion, as long as one less chicken dies for the sake of our appetites, then it's all good. I don't have time (or the desire) to make my own tofu, grow my own wheatgrass or prepare everything straight-from-the-earth-to-the-table. And I definitely don't have the time or desire (much less the skill) to prepare beautiful culinary works of art made from the most rare organic ingredients. Now don't get me wrong, I enjoy those things, and at least half of our meals are always full of raw organic fruits and vegetables, but everything we make is at a level that even a novice in the kitchen can do, and best of all we have saved you a lot time and trial and error figuring out how to make tofu interesting!

Think about our approach as Vegetarianism 101. It may suit you and it may not. But if you are still eating meat and most of your meals come in a bag or a box, you may want to start here. Trust me, it really is that easy. Even my son used our cookbook when he went off to college and has been cooking ever since (he's really good too!). If he can do it, you can too! As far as I'm concerned, any approach that helps people transition away from animal foods is a good one so we are humbly offering our approach and hope that it resonates with you or someone you may know.

Types of Vegetarians

Now may be a good time to clarify the definition of a vegetarian, since this terms has gotten watered down as of late. For example, I have a girlfriend that proudly announced to me recently that she is now vegan, because she only eats chicken and fish! So obviously, there is some confusion out there. Here's our attempt at shedding some light on the subject.

A vegetarian is someone who doesn't consume meat, poultry, pork, fish or seafood. Technically, there are three types of vegetarians; *lacto vegetarians*, *lacto-ovo vegetarians*, and *vegans*. Vegans are sometimes also referred to as "strict" vegetarians. *Lacto vegetarians* include dairy products in their diet, but do not eat eggs or anything that contains eggs or animal rennet.[1] *Lacto-ovo vegetarians* include dairy products and eggs in their diet. *Vegans* do not consume animal products of any kind, including butter and honey, and many vegans do not wear leather or fur.

Some people who eat fish still consider themselves to be vegetarians. In our opinion, and by the strictest definitions, people who eat fish or seafood are not considered to be vegetarians. As my daughter likes to say, "What plant do fish come from?"

My family and I are lacto-vegetarians, but 95% of the time we follow a vegan diet. In fact, this book and our other two, *Throwin' Down Vegetarian Style (Second Edition)*, and *Meatless Mondays: 52 Weeks of Meat-Free Meals* have recipes that are completely vegan. We believe in the merits of the vegan diet – ethically, nutritionally, and environmentally and have updated our recipes to reflect that.

So the question now is – what do we eat? It's easier for me to reiterate what we don't eat – meat, chicken, fish, eggs, and for the most part, dairy. That's it. Just five things. Other than that, we probably eat just like anyone else. There are literally thousands of things to eat that are healthful,

---

[1] *Animal rennet is obtained from the stomachs of young mammals. In most cases the source is from the lining of young calves. Rennet is used in most cheeses as an enzyme in the cheese hardening process. Many lacto vegetarians do not eat cheeses that contain animal rennet or animal enzymes. Many organic cheeses are made from vegetable enzymes and are suitable for these vegetarians. Normally, if the source of the enzymes is vegetarian, it will be noted in the list of ingredients.*

delicious, and nutritious that do not fall in into one of those five categories. For some reason, everyone thinks that just because you are vegetarian that you do not like hearty or flavorful food or that all you eat are alfalfa sprouts and carrots. This is not the case for us at all. We eat more than just salads and pasta. We even eat sweets and fried foods; we just make sure that they are vegetarian and are prepared in a healthy manner *(case in point- have you seen the photo of the Vegan Carrot Cake? – its soooo good!)*.

How to use this Quick Start Kit

We have designed this booklet to give you enough tools, information and resources to help you get started on your vegetarian path, whether it is a full time commitment or just an occasional break from meat. As the title indicates, we have provided 7 days of vegan dishes as well as a *Vegetarian Shopping Guide* and *Easy Transition Tips* to give you a head start. We also encourage you to review the other books and websites in the *Vegetarian Resources* section. There is a ton of useful information that is invaluable!

Finally, please visit our website at *www.21stCenturyVegetarians.com* for even more recipes and to join our mailing list or connect with us via various social networks to stay updated on the latest information in the vegetarian community. After you jump in and start your new way of eating, please send me feedback! You can email me directly at Martha@21stCenturyVegetarians.com. Enjoy!

Your choice of diet can influence your long term health prospects more than any other action you might take.

-Former U.S. Surgeon General C. Everett Koop

2

Top Five Reasons to be a Vegetarian

There are so many positive reasons to be a vegetarian that I could devote an entire book solely to that topic. But all it takes is *one* reason to make a change for a lifetime, as it did with our family. This is my "Top Five List" – hopefully you'll find one or two that are compelling enough to encourage you to make a change or at least consider this lifestyle. If you want more reasons, I encourage you to check out Pamela Rice's *101 Reasons Why I'm a Vegetarian*, from the Viva Vegie Society at www.vivavegie.org.

Reason #1 – Ethical Reasons

Over 10 billon animals are slaughtered each year in the most cruel, inhumane manner imaginable. These are living, breathing creatures who can feel fear, terror, and pain, just like humans can. In my opinion, this is a spiritual dichotomy. Few would argue that all spiritual paths promote tenets of peace, love and compassion for others and their suffering. If you do your own independent research on the great spiritual leaders and philosophers of the past and present, you will note that they, by an overwhelming majority, have adopted a non-violence creed, most notably one of vegetarianism. How then, can we proclaim to be truly seeking spirituality and sincerely following a spiritual path, if, on a daily basis every time we eat, we actually contribute to the suffering of so many of God's creatures? Is it that the thought of what we eat, and the journey the food takes on its way to our plate never even crosses our mind? Or, as the book *Why We Love Dogs, Eat Pigs, and Wear Cows: An Introduction to Carnism*, by Melanie Joy, PhD, asks - why do we put dogs or cats higher on the "emotional ladder" than cows, pigs, chickens, or fish?

Perhaps it is because most of us do not eat (or even live) in a conscious or mindful manner. Or specifically, perhaps we consider the animals we eat to be beasts and worthy of slaughter because they cannot talk or show emotions in the same manner as humans. Using that logic, the same would be true of our babies and young children, because although they cannot reason or even talk, there is no question that they can suffer.

As long as man continues to be the ruthless destroyer of lower living beings, he will never know health or peace. For as long as men massacre animals, they will kill each other. Indeed, he who sows the seeds of murder and pain cannot reap joy and love.

Pythagoras,
Greek Philosopher

This reminds me of a quote by philosopher Jeremy Bentham regarding the treatment of animals and their use for food; he states, *"The question is not 'Can they reason?' nor 'Can they talk?' but 'Can they suffer?"* Obviously, ALL creatures can suffer and there is no excuse – for convenience or otherwise – to cause unnecessary suffering if you consider yourself to be a proponent of peaceful and compassionate living. To illustrate this point further, Author Ellen G. White (1827 – 1915), in her book *The Ministry of Healing*, states:

"Flesh food is injurious to health, and whatever affects the body has a corresponding effect on the mind and the soul. Think of the cruelty to animals that meat eating involves, and its effect on those who inflict and those who behold it. How it destroys the tenderness with which we should regard those creatures of God!

"What man with a human heart, who has ever cared for domestic animals, could look into their eyes, so full of confidence and affection, and willingly give them over to the butcher's knife? How could he devour their flesh as a sweet morsel?"

So I leave you with this thought - what better way to affirm a peaceful and compassionate life choice every day, other than by what you eat?

Reason #2 – Vegetarians are Nine Times Less Likely to be Overweight than Non-Vegetarians

You'd pretty much have to be living under a rock if you don't know that obesity is now the number one health crisis in the United States. According to the American Obesity Association (AOA), (www.obesity.org), 66.3% of adult Americans (about 200 million), and 20% of children are categorized as being overweight or obese. For my demographic, African American women, that number climbs to 78%. That's nearly four of every five Black women! Each year, obesity and obesity related diseases cause at least 300,000 excess deaths in the United States, and the healthcare costs of American adults who are obese amount to approximately $147 billion. Obesity is now an epidemic in our country and is the root cause of many of the other diseases we suffer as a nation.

Obesity is the most prevalent, fatal, chronic, relapsing disorder of the 21st century. Obesity is a leading cause of United States mortality, morbidity, disability, healthcare utilization and healthcare costs. It is likely that the increase in obesity will strain our healthcare system with millions of additional cases of diabetes, heart disease and disability.

American Obesity Association

In September 2010, a study was conducted by the Organization for Economic Cooperation and Development which stated that three out of four Americans (75%) will be overweight or obese by 2020 (just ten years away!), and that disease rates and health care spending will balloon, unless governments, individuals and industry cooperate on a comprehensive strategy to combat the epidemic. The Paris-based organization, which brings together 33 of the world's leading economies, is better known for forecasting deficit and employment levels but the economic cost of excess weight — in health care, and in lives cut short and resources wasted — is a growing concern for many governments. According to the OECD, the lifespan of an obese person is up to 8-10 years shorter than that of a normal-weight person, the same loss of lifespan incurred by smoking.

In spite of all of the advancements we have made as a species, whether in the medical field, education, health and welfare, or otherwise, physically, we are in the worst shape of our lives. On average, Americans are 30% heavier than we were just one generation ago. A big factor in this is the type of food that we eat and the way in which it is processed and prepared.

The consumption of an animal-based diet is largely to blame for this condition, as well as many other diseases. Animal foods are far less healthy than they were just a generation ago due to the many chemicals, bacteria, growth hormones, and antibiotics that are common in the meat producing industry. The flesh of the animal foods we consume are saturated with these chemicals and are, in turn, ingested by us. How can we not suffer the consequences? We are literally becoming as large and unhealthy as the cows, chickens and pigs that we are eating.

Reason #3 – Vegetarians are Less Likely to Suffer From Heart Disease and Cancer

According to the American Heart Association, vegetarians have a lower risk of obesity, coronary heart disease, high blood pressure, diabetes, and some forms of cancer. Again, these ailments are all diet related. In March 2009, the Washington Post released a story, *Dying for some red meat? You May Be*, which states that:

> Eating red meat increases the chances of dying prematurely, according to a large federal study offering powerful new evidence that a diet that regularly includes steaks, burgers and pork chops is hazardous to your health.

> The study of more than 500,000 middle-age and elderly Americans found that those who consumed the equivalent of about a small hamburger every day were more than 30% more likely to die during the 10 years they were followed, mostly from heart disease and cancer. Sausage, cold cuts and other processed meats increased the risk too.

Supporting these findings with even more comprehensive research, The New York Times Bestseller *The China Study*, by T. Colin Campbell, details the connection between nutrition and heart disease, diabetes and cancer and also its ability to reduce or reverse the risk or effects of these deadly illnesses. According to Dr. Campbell, *"People who ate the most animal-based foods got the most chronic disease ... People who ate the most plant-based foods were the healthiest and tended to avoid chronic disease. These results could not be ignored."*

In my opinion, The China Study is a must-read book for *everyone* because it cuts through the haze of misinformation and delivers an insightful message to anyone living with cancer, diabetes, heart disease, obesity, and those concerned with the effects of aging.

Reason #4 – Vegetarians Have a Significantly Lower Risk of Diabetes

No surprise, but this is again linked to Reason #2. Specifically, vegetarians are half as likely to suffer from Type 2 Diabetes as non-vegetarians. Why do we care? We hear a lot about diabetes these days, but do you really know the consequences? Why do we care? Why is diabetes so dangerous? According to a recent report issued by the State of California and the Governor's Summit on Health, Nutrition and Obesity, some of the gravest effects of diabetes are:

- Diabetes damages organs, destroys cells, and shortens lives
- Diabetes is now the sixth leading cause of death in the United States
- Men who become diabetic by age 40 will lose more than 11 years of life, and women who become diabetic by age 40 will lose more than 14 years
- Diabetes increases the risk for heart disease six-fold, and multiplies the risk of stroke by four
- One dollar out of every seven spent on health care in this country is for diabetes treatment
- Each year in the U.S., 24,000 people will go blind, 28,000 will experience kidney failure, and 82,000 will have amputations – all as a direct result of diabetes.

That's the bad news. The good news is that Type 2 diabetes in most cases is completely manageable and at many times even preventable by:

- Maintaining a healthy weight
- Increasing fruit and vegetable consumption
- Increasing fiber intake
- Decreasing fat intake, and
- Increasing physical exercise.

A vegetarian diet addresses the first four of the five actions above. As mentioned before, vegetarians are nine times less likely to be overweight or obese than non-vegetarians and plant based foods are naturally higher in fiber, lower in fat, and contain NO cholesterol.

My family and I know up close and personal how ravaging the effects of diabetes are. My mother, who will turn 80 this year, has suffered from obesity, heart disease, high cholesterol, and diabetes for the past 20 – 30 years. Each year, she degenerates more and more, as she is now at the point where she can no longer care for herself, and do even simple things such as cook, climb stairs, or even shower without assistance. Earlier this year, things got so bad that it looked as though my sister and I were going to have to put her in assisted living, something we did not want to do, but her weight had ballooned to over 270 pounds and her blood sugar and blood pressure were completely out of control. As a last ditch effort, we decided to move her close to me, and put her on a completely vegetarian diet – nothing strict, just the same meals my family and I eat.

"Growing old does not make us sick...it's growing sick that makes us old!"

Baroness Benita von Klingspor, author

The results were amazing. In less than two months, she lost over 35 pounds, was able to eliminate injectable insulin (previously she was taking 3 to 4 shots a day), was able to eliminate her cholesterol medication and reduce her blood pressure medication because her cholesterol and blood pressure were within normal range when she went in for her next checkup. Her doctor was in shock. He said he had never seen such a dramatic turnaround in a woman of her age, and asked what my secret was. You already know the answer to that.....

Reason #5 – Vegetarian Diets Will Help Save Our Planet!

In 2003, the Johns Hopkins University Bloomberg School of Public Health started an initiative called "Meatless Monday" (www.MeatlessMonday.com) with the goal of reducing meat consumption by 15% to improve public health and the health of our planet. Even if you are not fully vegetarian, if everyone in the United States adopted a vegetarian diet *just one day per week* (surely we can do that!), consider these environmental benefits:

> *"Nothing will benefit human health and increase chances for survival of life on earth as much as the evolution to a vegetarian diet."*
>
> Albert Einstein

- *Conserve Fuel* - of all the raw materials and fossil fuels used in the United States, more than one-third are used to raise animals for food. Factory Farming is the largest contributor to greenhouse gasses in the United States. *Not eating meat one day per week would save 12 BILLION GALLONS of gasoline a year* and result in a greenhouse gas reduction equivalent as if everyone in the U.S. drove Toyota Prius hybrid car.

- *Conserve Water Resources* – nearly half of all the water consumed in the United States is used to raise animals for food. It takes 2500 gallons of water to produce a pound of meat, but only 25 gallons to produce a pound of wheat. A totally vegetarian diet requires 300 gallons of water per day, while a meat-based diet requires more than 4,000 gallons of water per day. It takes 5 times as much water to produce meat as it does to produce other high protein vegetarian options. *The amount of water required to produce a 5.2 oz. hamburger is the equivalent of taking a four-hour shower*. Eliminating meat once a week would save a tremendous amount of water.

- *Reduce Pollution* – farmed animals produce 130 times as much excrement as the entire human population of the United States.

According to the EPA, the run-off from factory farms pollutes our rivers and lakes more than all other industrial sources combined. A 15% reduction in pollution would make a HUGE impact on our environment.

- ***Slow Global Warming*** - Livestock production is a major cause of deforestation, thus a major source of global warming, hoarding 30 percent of the land surface of the planet. Livestock production is responsible for 18% of the greenhouse gas emissions. Vehicles are only 13%. Going meatless even one day per week will help slow the growth of global warming.

So here's the bottom line - given all of the factors mentioned above, in addition to many others, surely you can adopt a meatless diet just one day a week, right? Why not join millions of others, including major school districts such as the Baltimore and Washington, D.C. public school districts, and numerous colleges and universities such as Syracuse University, Vassar College, Carnegie Mellon University, UC Santa Cruz and many more in "Meatless Monday." For a list of school districts, celebrities, chefs, political leaders, and more that have taken the pledge to go meatless one day a week, visit *www.meatlessmonday.com/whos-going-meatless*. If you need some help getting started, be sure to check out our book, *Meatless Mondays: 52 Weeks of Meat-Free Meals* for a year's worth of vegetarian recipes!

A human can be healthy without killing animals for food. Therefore if he eats meat he participates in taking animal life merely for the sake of his appetite.

-Leo Tolstoy

3

Vegetarian Myths – The Truth Revealed!

T his is one of my favorite topics – vegetarian myths! I *so* enjoy dispelling the myths about vegetarian living – it's amazing how many urban legends there are floating around out there. Over the past 25 years I believe I have heard them all. According to most of these myths, by now I should be weak, malnourished or even dead. Happily, the truth is just the opposite – my entire family is strong, healthy, and very much alive – even my grown children! I am not claiming to be a medical or nutritional expert, but I am an expert at raising a healthy family. As you can see from our pictures, especially of my kids who have been vegetarian since birth, we are not lacking strength, stamina, or good health. As

> *A misconception remains a misconception even when it is shared by a majority of the people.*
>
> Author Unknown

you read this chapter I encourage you to have an open mind, consider the information I've presented, but don't just take my word for it - do your own research! You will be amazed that the answers are there in plain sight, you just have to wade through the misinformation that is being driven primarily by the quest for corporate profits. Don't be a slave to the system – use your power of intellect and reason to make better choices for yourself and your family. You can be vegetarian and be completely healthy – in fact even healthier than most meat eaters.

And now for the number one question.....

Where Do You Get Your Protein?

I absolutely positively guarantee that at least 95% of people ask me this question as soon as they learn that I am vegetarian. The other 5% say something like, *"I used to be a vegetarian but I had to go back to eating meat because I wasn't getting enough protein."* Basically, Americans have an obsession with protein consumption – an obsession created by the meat and dairy industries that have been brainwashing us right into the worst health in the history of mankind. This obsession is matched in magnitude only by misunderstanding. Therefore, what you end up with is a society that is obsessed with something that they completely misunderstand. That's not a good combination!

The truth is that not only do we get adequate protein but my family and I probably get *MORE protein* on a daily basis than the average meat eater. The difference is that my family and I eat a variety of products from various parts of the plant kingdom which are not only extremely high in protein but are much higher quality, and are proteins that are more easily assimilated than that from animal sources.

How's that for a myth buster? Not convinced? Take a look at the chart on the next page, **PROTEIN COMPARISON CHART – SORTED BY PROTEIN LEVELS**. No, your eyes are not deceiving you. The top five sources of protein on this chart are completely vegan – from plant sources only. This is where my family gets their protein – from these sources directly or from products made from these sources. So, as you can see, if we eat a balanced diet incorporating plant based protein sources, there is no way we can have a deficiency. And, when I say "better protein" it is because vegan proteins are completely free of cholesterol and uric acid which are two components in meat that are widely linked to chronic diseases.

PROTEIN COMPARISON CHART - SORTED BY PROTEIN LEVELS

	Description	Amount	Protein (grams)	Cholesterol (milligrams)	Fat (grams)	Fiber (grams)	Calories
Vegan	Wheat Gluten (aka Seitan)	approx 1 cup	75	0	2	1	370
Vegan	Soybeans	1 cup	68	0	37	17	830
Vegan	Lentils (raw)	1 cup	50	0	2	59	678
Vegan	Kidney Beans	1 cup	44	0	1	46	607
Vegan	Black Beans	1 cup	42	0	3	30	662
	Tuna, canned	4 oz	30	35	9	0	210
	Ground Beef Patties	4oz patty	26	95	27	0	333
Vegan	Peanut Butter, chunky	1/3 cup	24	0	50	8	589
	Salmon	4 oz	23	62	15	0	235
	Steak, Porterhouse	4 oz	23	64	17	0	252
Vegan	Tofu, raw, firm	approx 1/2 cup	20	0	11	3	183
Vegan	Tempeh	approx 1/2 cup	19	0	11	?	193
	Chicken - uncooked	1/2 breast	18	56	8	0	150
	Ham, deli slices	4 slices	18	64	10	2	183
	Turkey Breast	4 slices	14	36	1	0	87
	Eggs, whole raw	2 eggs	13	423	10	0	143
	Bacon	4 slices	11	62	34	0	351
Vegan	Walnuts	1/2 cup	9	0	38	4	383
Vegan	Brown Rice, cooked	1 cup	5	0	2	4	216

SOURCE: USDA FOOD NUTRITION INFORMATION (www.nal.usda.gov/fnic/foodcomp/search/)
Copyright © 2009 Martha Theus

It should also be noted that all sources of animal protein (including fish and eggs) contain cholesterol and have little or no fiber. No sources of plant protein contain cholesterol and most have substantial amounts of fiber, since plants are primarily fibrous foods. According to the American Heart Association, (Americanheart.org) two of the most important factors for lowering your risk of heart disease, in addition to maintaining a healthy weight, are to reduce your cholesterol intake (to less than 200mg/day) and increase your fiber intake (at least 25 – 30g/day).

In 2003, a comprehensive study conducted by the American Dietary Association (ADA) concluded that a vegetarian based diet was as sufficient in nutrients as an animal based diet, and was actually healthier in all major categories. For example, did you know that consuming an excess amount of animal protein can actually lead to symptoms associated with kidney disease and osteoporosis? Too much animal protein can leech your bones of calcium, thus resulting in osteoporosis. In addition, if the body takes in more animal protein than it needs, the excess can be deposited into the kidneys and can lead to kidney disease. This study also noted that:

- Vegetarians had lower rates of cardiovascular disease primarily due to the fact that non-animal foods are completely free of cholesterol, the leading cause of heart disease.
- Vegetarians also have lower rates of colon cancer because they do not eat meat and according to the ADA, both red and white meats have been independently linked to an increased risk of colon cancer.
- Excess consumption of dairy products and calcium have been linked to an increased risk for prostate cancer.
- Vegetarians are half as likely to suffer from gallstones, rheumatoid arthritis, and even dementia (Alzheimer's disease), all of which have been linked to meat based diets.

See what I mean when I say that that we not only get enough protein, but *better* protein? Convinced? If not, consider this: if you think it is impossible for vegetarians to get enough protein then how do you explain that some of the largest, most powerful animals on earth are in fact vegetarian? Have you considered that most animals that are eaten are vegetarians themselves? So, in effect, isn't eating meat just eating recycled vegetables that are pumped up with hormones, chemicals, and other unsavory things? So, now that I have answered the question "where do you get your protein?" let me ask you the same thing, "Where do you get *your* protein?"

One farmer says to me, "You cannot live on vegetable food solely, for it furnishes nothing to make the bones with;" and so he religiously devotes a part of his day to supplying himself with the raw material of bones; walking all the while he talks behind his oxen, which, with vegetable-made bones, jerk him and his lumbering plow along in spite of every obstacle.

Henry David Thoreau, *Walden*

No Meat? Now What?

Let's say you're interested in giving up meat either for a day or a lifetime. Your next question may be exactly the same as mine was 25 years ago – *"No Meat? Now What?"* When I went from eating pork chops to a vegetarian in the course of one day, I really could not imagine a meal that was not centered around meat. But where there's a will, there's a way, and that is far more true today than it was in 1985. Back then was like living in the dark ages – no internet, no resource groups, and no Whole Foods Markets (at least not in my neighborhood)! We were completely on our own so I did the only thing I knew to do which was start with my Mother's recipes and remake them in a more healthful vegetarian manner. I became a big fan of the mock meats since they seemed "familiar" and were so easy to prepare. But along the way I also learned the advantages of eating whole foods, raw fruits and vegetables, and many varieties of nuts, grains and legumes. It is not a question of what you can't eat – change your mind set to what you can eat and you will be amazed at the variety and choices all around you.

This book is intended to introduce you to a few of our favorite vegetarian products and give you a head start to broaden your perspective and knowledge base. A list of the products we use in the recipes presented can be found in *Chapter Five: Vegetarian Products Guide*. Please note that this is a very short list – we don't want to overwhelm you in your first week. A more comprehensive list can be found in our other two books, *Throwin' Down Vegetarian Style! (Second Edition)* and *Meatless Mondays: 52 Weeks of Meat-Free Meals*. To get started, if you try a few of these products and recipes, pretty soon you will see delicious, healthy vegetarian options everywhere. That's how it is when Kamaal and I go shopping now – we really don't even see the meat – all we see are dozens of new things that we have not tried or that we can convert into a great new vegetarian dish.

Isn't It Expensive and Inconvenient?

Other than the misconception that vegetarians do not get enough protein, I would say that this is the second-most widespread untruth – that eating a healthy vegetarian diet every day is expensive and inconvenient. First of all, it depends on how you define "expensive and inconvenient." Everyone has their own interpretation of this, but it is all relative. For example, I don't know what I'll do if I see another overweight and obviously unhealthy sister get out of her $100,000 car while swinging her $1,200 weave and carrying her $800 purse walk into the nearest fast food joint because "it's cheaper and quicker than cooking at home." You may think I'm exaggerating, but trust me, I'm not. I see and hear this sort of thing *daily*. In fact, just recently I was at a book signing and met an African-American woman who was about my age (late forties) who fell into the 78% overweight category that I mentioned in the previous chapter. We were talking about my book and my approach to maintaining a healthy vegetarian lifestyle. She was intrigued - enough to buy the book - but then gave me the following reasons why she did not feel it would be possible for her; 1) it was too expensive, 2) she did not have time to cook - even though she was single and had no children - and 3) it was too inconvenient.

I've heard these same "protests" hundreds of times and yet the hypocrisy never ceases to amaze me. In this same conversation (which we continued into the parking lot), she told me about how she has some sort of special weave process done to her hair in a salon in Beverly Hills which takes hours and costs about $1,200 every two months (I have to admit – her hair was whipped!), and that she eats out because she does not have time to cook, and that even if she did she could not afford to eat organic because the prices are so high. By the time she finished talking, we had arrived at her car. A shiny, brand new Lexus.....the same one I have on my vision board which I'm sure is on its way to me but has not yet manifested! In my first book, *Throwin' Down Vegetarian Style!* (First Edition), I made a point that most people take better care of their cars than they do their own bodies. For women, I would have to say that they take better care of their hair and their cars than they do themselves.

But this is not about my opinion. Let's look at the facts. On the subject of this lifestyle being too expensive, allow me to shed some light on the truth. I am still a practicing Certified Public Accountant, so in addition to keeping my client's books balanced to the penny; I do the same for our household also. Seriously – *to the penny.* Every dime that flows through our house is accounted for, assigned to the proper category, and reconciled. I do monthly financial statements at home just as I do for my clients, so I know exactly what I spend on groceries and eating out. Each month, we spend an average of $1,200 - $1,500/month on groceries and related household items such as toiletries, paper products, laundry supplies, etc. Even if we take the highest number, $1,500, that breaks down to $50/day for a family of five (two grown men, and three grown women - my mother is included since we prepare all of her meals). This is $10/day per person for ALL of our food and various toiletries and household items. With this, we eat 100% vegetarian organic food three times per day. This breaks down to just over $3/meal per person. A far as eating out goes, we spend less that $100/month for all five of us. Not that we have anything against eating out, it's just that we honestly prefer home cooked food filled with love over restaurant food that is usually full of addictive elements such as sugar, fat, and salt.

If you really keep track of what you spend on food for even just one week, I am positive that you'll find you can eat much better if you take a little time to prepare healthy food at home. Try it – track all of your food spending (Starbucks, vending machines, lunch trucks, Subway, grocery stores, etc.) and see if it doesn't come to more than $10/day. I have friends that start each morning off at Starbucks, and by the time they get a latte, a pastry, and leave a tip, they are already at $8 and haven't even had a full meal yet! Whereas for that same $8 (or $10 if I'm splurging), I enjoy three full vegan organic meals – prepared at home and with love and care.

Bottom line, it is not more expensive to eat vegetarian organic food when you compare it to what most Americans are doing which is stuffing themselves with poor quality fast food under the guise that it is cheaper and more convenient. Speaking of convenience, for the past 25 years I have cooked every day for my family (unless we have leftovers from the previous day). Kamaal helps me now but regardless of who does what, all meals for all five of us are prepared daily. When I tell people this, they look at me as though I'm crazy and immediately protest that they do not have time for that. When I ask, "do you have time to eat?' of course the answer is "Yes!' My response is, "then you have time to cook!" With just a little bit of forethought and planning, I can prepare enough food for the day for all five of us in under an hour – *always*. Vegetarian food is much quicker to prepare because the food is inherently safer – no blood, bacteria or other harmful things that you have to literally cook to death.

Think about how long it really takes when you eat out. First of all, at best, you have to drive to the drive-thru, place your order, and then wait. Rarely can you do that in less than 20 minutes total. Or, perhaps you don't live on fast food (good for you!), but instead you eat at higher-end establishments where you actually sit down and have your order taken. In this case, including travel time, you are talking about at least an hour. How many times a day or week do you do this? How about everyone in your family? The time really does add up. Due to the lack of some very basic planning and organization, most people rely on complete strangers to provide a very intimate service for us – preparation of the food which will literally become a part of our very flesh and blood. Do you really want to give a complete stranger that much power on a daily basis? Who knows what is actually in that food and who knows what they are doing to it? Do you really think that is a good way to eat, day in and day out?

I guarantee that not only in the long run, but even right now, on a daily basis, it is quicker, cheaper, and healthier to eat organic vegetarian food prepared at home. Just try it for a week using some of my simple recipes and you'll see that it's true! Not to mention that in the long run you will definitely see the benefits. As I said before, we spend $1,200 - $1,500/month on food for the five of us; this our largest *investment* (not expense) other than our housing cost. In other words, our grocery bill is higher than all of our other expenses – car – entertainment – utilities, etc. But isn't that how it should be? There is no way, in good conscious, I could rationalize spending more money on a car, clothes, weave, or even a house at the expense of caring for the only body that the Lord has given me. We have been given something priceless - a body that houses and transports our spirits - so that we may live the most abundant life possible and hopefully help others and make the world a better place in our own way. Our bodies have the amazing ability to repair and heal themselves if we take the time and effort to learn about how they function and how to keep them in the best shape. Yet as I said before it is far too common to see an unhealthy person in a $100,000 car in the drive-thru window purchasing a $4.99 meal full of processed, poor quality ingredients that can barely pass for food. Would you put sugar, fat and salt in the gas tank of your luxury car? Would you wash your hair (whether it is natural or a $1,200 weave) with any random brand of dish soap that happens to be on sale? Then why would you do the equivalent to your body? In the long run, if you continue to do so it will be far more expensive – in health care costs and lost productivity. When you are too sick to even leave the house or take a walk with someone you love, there is no car, house, or hairstyle that will ease that pain. Ultimately, it is usually a matter of priorities, not finances. When you look in the mirror, your priorities are reflected back to you. Do you like what you see?

Let food be thy medicine and medicine be thy food.

-Hippocrates (460 B.C.)

A journey of a thousand miles begins with a single step.

Lao-tzu, Chinese philosopher (604 BC - 531 BC)

4

Easy Transition Tips

There are so many ways to approach a transition to a vegetarian or vegan diet. This book represents our family's process which may or may not be suitable for you. In addition to what I've presented here, please check out the *Vegetarian Resources* section at the end of this book for more ideas from other authors, businesses, and health professionals. For those of you who want to jump in right away, I have delineated our process into the following easy tips – converting meals, preparing food, shopping, and eating out.

Convert Your Favorite Meals

The simplest way, in my opinion, to convert to a vegetarian diet is to pick a few of your favorite meals, and find the comparable products to make it vegetarian. *(This is also the best way to proceed if you are trying to ease your family into it! By all means, do not do anything too wild or drastic – you may only have one chance to get them to "buy in"!)* For example, if you make an awesome meat lasagna, just use "Boca Crumbles" by Boca Burger® in place of ground beef. Everything else should be the same except for the fact that when you sauté the Boca Crumbles they will be done in 5 minutes instead of the 20 or 30 minutes it takes to cook real ground beef. In addition, virtually any type of chicken dish can be made with Gardein® instead of actual chicken. Just remember not to cook the vegetarian products as long as you would actual meat – remember, most of these products can be eaten raw or with very little cooking because there is no blood, bacteria, etc. in them. The only reason most need to be cooked at all is simply to change the texture somewhat and to blend in any added spices or sauces. Pretty much just like you would cook meat, right? Very rarely do you get a package of chicken or meat and eat it raw. Of course you have to season it and cook it for the appropriate amount of time so that it is prepared to your liking. Get the idea? It's really just that simple.

One footnote I would add to this section is this – if your favorite meals are not necessarily healthy, use this opportunity to start introducing healthier habits. For example, as I noted previously, our family eats lots of raw, organic fruits and vegetables – normally half of our meals consist of a large vegetable or fruit salad. I cannot stress enough the importance of raw foods and of organic foods. Even I had to learn this since the publication of our first book back in 2007 – since then, and thanks to so many of our readers and our own independent research, we have incorporated a lot more raw foods into our daily meals and we can tell the difference! Try to make sure that at least half your plate is filled with nutritious, vibrant raw foods before eating your cooked options.

Prepare and Pack Your Food

I find that this is the one area where people get "stuck" so if you can master this, you've got it made. As I said in the previous chapters, whenever I tell someone that I (or my daughter Kamaal) cook every day, they look at me either in awe or like I'm crazy. The reality is that we as a people have become so disconnected with our bodies that we cannot even *eat* without someone feeding us. Does that make sense? Isn't it time to get back to basics and learn to feed ourselves and our families again?

Once you get into a routine, it is actually very simple. I never spend more than 45 minutes to an hour *a day* preparing food for our entire family of five. The benefits of eating your own, home cooked food are endless, including:

1) Eating home cooked food is less expensive,
2) Eating home cooked food is normally more nutritious
3) Eating home cooked food may help you lose weight *(most restaurants want to get you "hooked" and create a "sensual" experience when you eat so the food is often filled with sugar, fat and salt).*
4) Eating home cooked food is filled with your love and vibrations, not the vibrations of a perfect stranger earning minimum wage!

Don't get me wrong, I have nothing against eating out, but my family and I treat eating out as a form of entertainment, just as we treat going to the movies or the theatre. I enjoy eating out very much just like I enjoy going to the movies but I would never do either three times a day. Get the point? Sure, treat yourself to a meal out every now and then but don't let things get to the point where you are so dependent upon restaurants that you literally will not eat unless eat out.

A few more things you can do to help with this part of your transition:

1) Buy Tupperware or some sort of food storage system that is portable for taking food to work or school.
2) Shred or chop large quantities of fresh vegetables and fruit at least twice a week and store them in your refrigerator. The concept is to have a "salad bar in your fridge" which will encourage you to eat enough raw foods.
3) Make large quantities of food (soup, rice dishes, etc.) that will keep well throughout the week.
4) Plan your meals for the next week and shop in advance so that you are not on a "scavenger hunt" every day for lunch or dinner.
5) Pick a slow day during the week or weekend to do most of your cooking or food preparation like the chopping, shredding, etc. You will be amazed at how much you can get done in just a couple of hours in the kitchen on the weekends. Better yet, if you have kids, get them involved too! The sooner they learn to nourish themselves the better!

How and Where To Shop

So many people approach vegetarian eating as something completely alien, so much so that they build up a resistance from the very beginning. If nothing else, the purpose of this book is to show you how EASY it is to live this lifestyle and that the few minor inconveniences are well worth the effort.

First of all, you have to know how and where to shop. Although a lot of the items I cook can be found in all chain groceries stores, I prefer going to markets that cater to healthier living and have more variety. Within three miles of my home, I have a Whole Foods Market, Trader Joes, Ralph's Grocery Store, Fresh and Easy Market, a local in-town grocery store, and two weekly farmer's markets. I admit, I am lucky to have these options so close to my home, but that was not always the case. We lived in Maryland a few years back and the closest Whole Foods Market and Trader Joes was over 20 miles away. That was no joke especially considering the inclement weather we had at times. Even still, I was able to find many options in my local grocery store – maybe just not all of my favorites.

Regardless of where you are accustomed to shopping, I would encourage you to check out your local farmer's market and your local store that carries health food. You will be amazed at the number of products that can easily replace whatever you are now using for meat or dairy. And please, don't get sticker shock! Pound for pound, or ounce for ounce, the prices will typically be higher but the quality is so much better. In addition, the government does not subsidize organic vegetarian food like it does the meat and dairy industry so please keep this in mind. The price of meat is actually much more than the price of vegetarian options, it's just that our tax dollars are underwriting much of this cost.

Finally, once you convert a few of your favorite meals, make a commitment to experiment with a new dish at least once a month so that things do not get routine. If you fall in love with a certain product and cannot find it in your local health food store, ask for it! I have had such success working with store managers in this way – in fact when I lived in Maryland I would get products by the case and so that most of my shopping was done once a month. Do your research, online and otherwise, and ask for what you need.

Eating Out and Traveling

I understand that many of you, for a variety of reasons, will still eat out on a regular basis. If you find yourself in this category, that's okay – you can still maintain a vegetarian diet. When I was working for a large international corporation in the Internal Audit Department I would have to travel for days on end and even though I would bring some food along with me, the international travel was a bit tricky due to agriculture restrictions so I had to eat many of my meals in restaurants. In reality, it was a nice break and a chance to try some local cuisine so I really did not mind. If you travel a lot or have such a hectic schedule that you can't prepare your food at home for a period of time, here are some tips:

1) Visit www.HappyCow.net for a domestic and international directory of vegetarian and vegetarian friendly restaurants and markets. This is absolutely, positively my favorite website for finding good restaurants – I have used it for over ten years and have found awesome spots to eat right here in Los Angeles and even in Central America and Europe. I also have their iPhone app- VegOut, which I use all the time.

2) If there are no vegetarian restaurants close to where you are, try a variety of ethnic restaurants knows for their fabulous vegetarian food such as Asian, Mediterranean, and Indian. In 2008, I spent most of the year on the road visiting the same city in Northern California for business. I always had a room with a microwave and a refrigerator, so I would stock up at Whole Foods Market or Trader Joes on the first night, and if I got bored I would supplement my meals by eating out at one of my favorite Thai, Lebanese, or Indian restaurants. Each one had awesome vegan options that tasted like authentic home cooked meals!

3) Even if you are "roughing it" on a long road trip or something, remember vegetarian food usually stays fresh longer than non-vegetarian food because by definition it is "cleaner" in that it does

not contain any blood, feces, etc. to turn rancid. My husband and I used to spend quite a bit of time on the road chasing my son around the country when he was playing basketball. We would always bring a cooler with fresh fruit and nuts for snacks, and also a few packages of vegetarian deli slices such as Tofurky® which we would slap on a veggie sub from Subway® or Quiznos® because they seemed to be at every rest stop. We even did that on a recent movie he shot in Fresno – I would buy two foot long veggie subs from Subway®, put sliced Tofurky® on each one, and then re-wrap them so he could have healthy vegan food on the set. It was cheap, good, nutritious and quite convenient!

I hope these tips have been helpful and you are inspired to jump in! Believe me, in the past 25 years I have been in so many situations – domestically and abroad – and have never had to compromise my commitment to vegetarianism. A way will always be made for you, especially when you make a step toward embracing a healthier, more compassionate way of eating. Have fun! I'm excited for you!

5

V

Vegetarian Shopping Guide

The products listed in this section are for the recipes I've provided in this book. Remember, this is a very short list and is not intended to be all encompassing. I don't want to present too much in this starter guide, because the entire point is to start with the simplest, most easily accessible items that also happen to be some of our favorites!

If you want more, please refer to one of our other books, *Meatless Mondays: 52 Weeks of Meat-Free Meals* which has over 52 vegan recipes, or *Throwin' Down Vegetarian Style!* (Second Edition) which has over 75 of our favorite vegan and vegetarian recipes. Both are available in paperback and eBook formats on our website at www.21stCenturyVegetarians.com.

Some things to remember – if you cannot find these items, ask! Most can be found in health food stores across the nation. I also encourage you to visit the related websites and contact the customer service departments to find out where these items are sold in your area.

7 DAY VEGETARIAN STARTER KIT — VEGETARIAN PRODUCT GUIDE		
PRODUCT, VENDOR, WEBSITE	RECIPE(S)	PHOTO
Seitan White Wave www.tofutown.net	Barbeque Seitan	
Tofurky® Italian Sausage Turtle Island Foods www.tofurkey.com	Vegan Deep Dish Pizza Penne Pasta with Italian Sausage	
Gardein® Garden Protein International www.gardein.com	Chik'n Tortilla Soup Fried Chik'n	
Smart Ground Mexican Style Veggie Crumbles Light Life www.lightlife.com	Enchiladas	
Tempeh – Organic Garden Veggie Light Life www.lightlife.com *(tempeh is very common – other brands are available also)*	Tempeh Tuna Wraps	

7 DAY VEGETARIAN STARTER KIT — VEGETARIAN PRODUCT GUIDE		
PRODUCT, VENDOR, WEBSITE	RECIPE(S)	PHOTO
Tofurky® Deli Slices –Hickory Smoked Turtle Island Foods www.tofurkey.com	Tofurky® Veggie Wraps	
Liquid Aminos Bragg Live Foods, Inc. www.bragg.com	Tempeh Tuna Wraps	
Miso Mayo – Spicy Red Pepper Flavor So Good Food Co www.misomayo.com	Tofurky® Veggie Wraps	
Vegenaise Follow Your Heart www.followyourheart.com	Tempeh Tuna Wraps Tofurky® Veggie Wraps	
Daiya Cheese, cheddar or mozzarella flavor Daiya Foods www.daiyafoods.com	Vegan Deep Dish Pizza Enchiladas	

7 DAY VEGETARIAN STARTER KIT — VEGETARIAN PRODUCT GUIDE		
PRODUCT, VENDOR, WEBSITE	RECIPE(S)	PHOTO
Spike® Seasoning Modern Products/Fern Natural Foods www.modernfern.com	Fried Chik'n Sautéed Tofu	
Vegan Cream Cheese – Plain Tofutti www.tofutti.com	Vegan Carrot Cake	
Silk Soy Milk White Wave Foods www.silksoymilk.com	Vegan Carrot Cake	
Silk French Vanilla Creamer White Wave Foods www.silksoymilk.com	Vegan Carrot Cake	
Earth Balance Natural Buttery Spread Earth Balance www.earthbalancenatural.com	Vegan Carrot Cake	

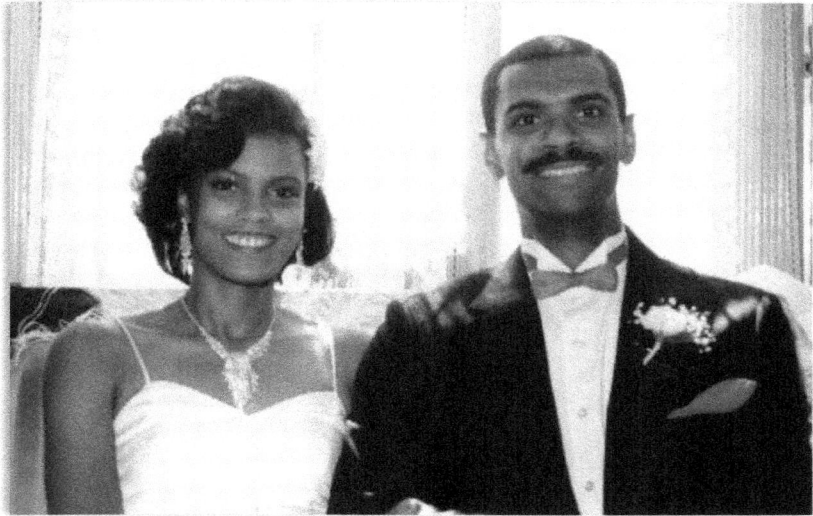

Above Photo:
Martha and Londale, September 1985.

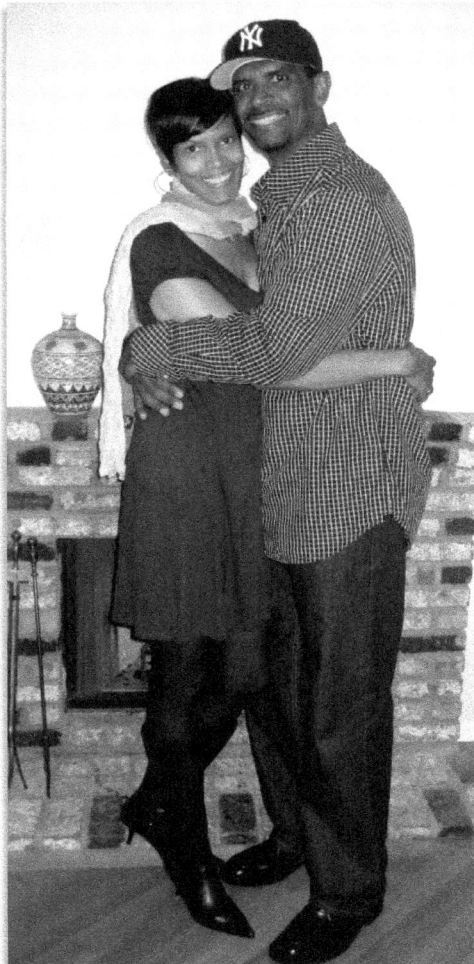

Left Photo:
Martha and Londale, September 2010. This month we celebrated our 25th wedding anniversary — hard to believe 25 years has passed so quickly! The fact that we have not visibly aged is a testament to our vegetarian lifestyle, and the fact that *"Black Don't Crack!"*

To see color photos, download the FREE eBook at:

www.21stCenturyVegetarians.com.

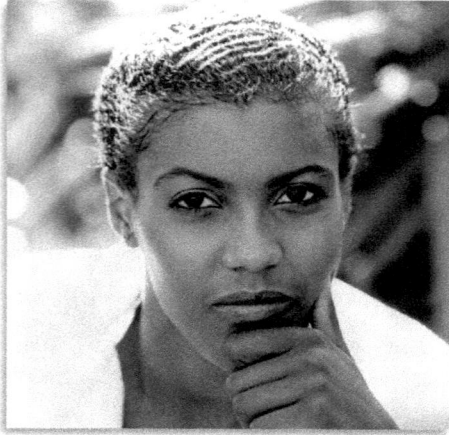

Martha, circa 1984

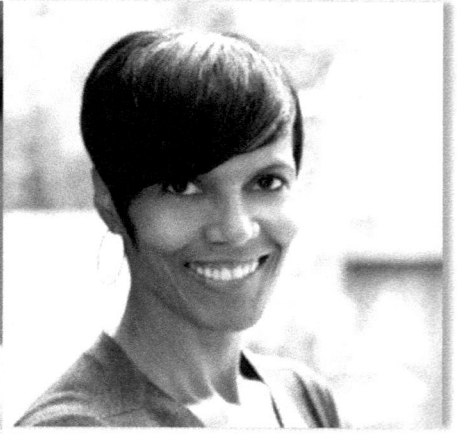

Martha 2010

Below: My Two Leading Men! Londale, Sr., 53 (left), Londale, Jr., 23 (right)

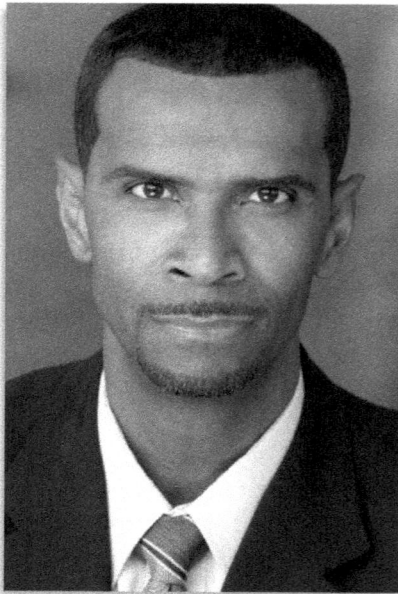

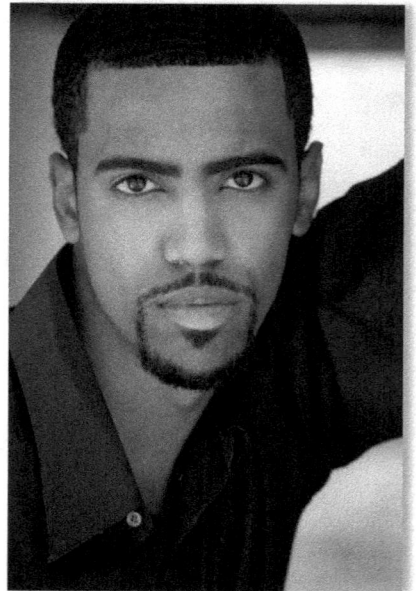

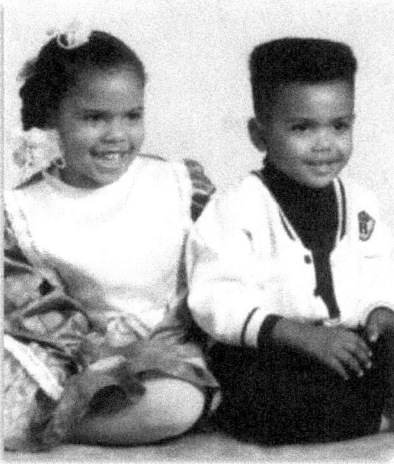

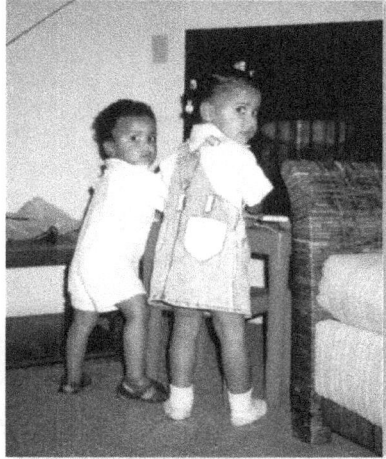

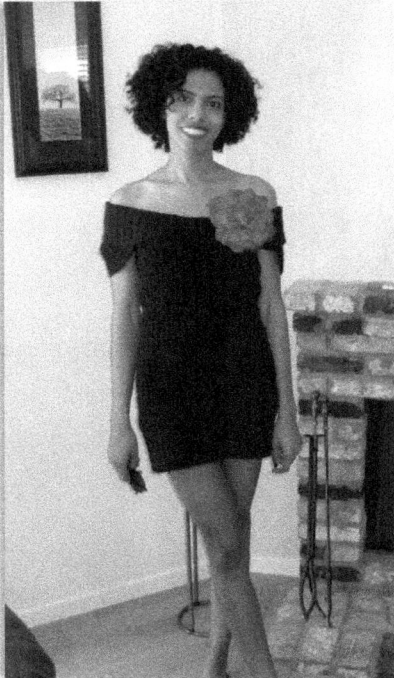

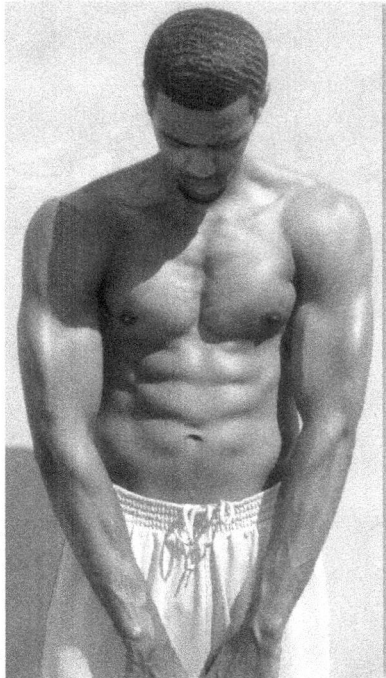

Upper Left and Right: My vegetarian babies! Kamaal and Londale — about 1989 and 1988, respectively.

Lower Left and Right: My vegetarian babies! (Yes — they are still my babies!). Kamaal and Londale — 2010 and 2009, respectively. Take a look at my baby boy — who said vegetarians can't build muscle?

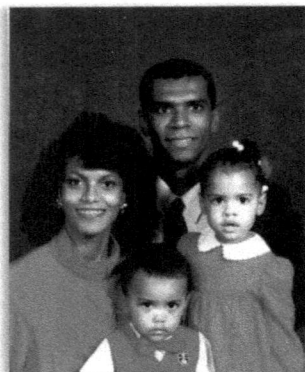

**Our Family throughout the years —
Martha, Londale Sr., Kamaal, Londale, Jr.**

Left: circa 1988 (you can tell it was the '80's because of my big hair!)

Middle: Maryland, 2006. *Photo by Kea Taylor*

Bottom: Los Angeles, 2010. *Photo by Brennen Scott*

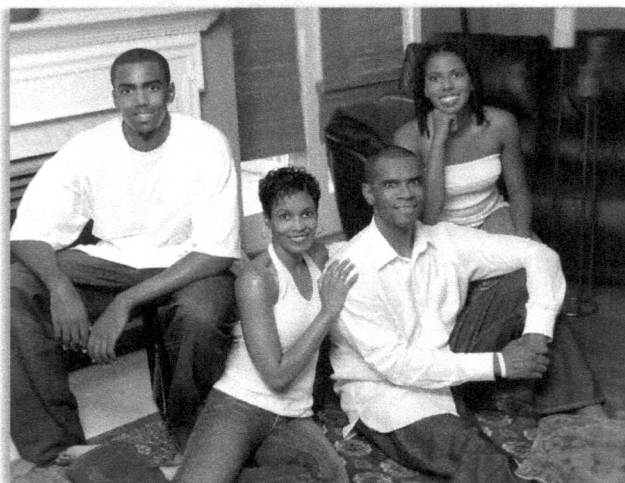

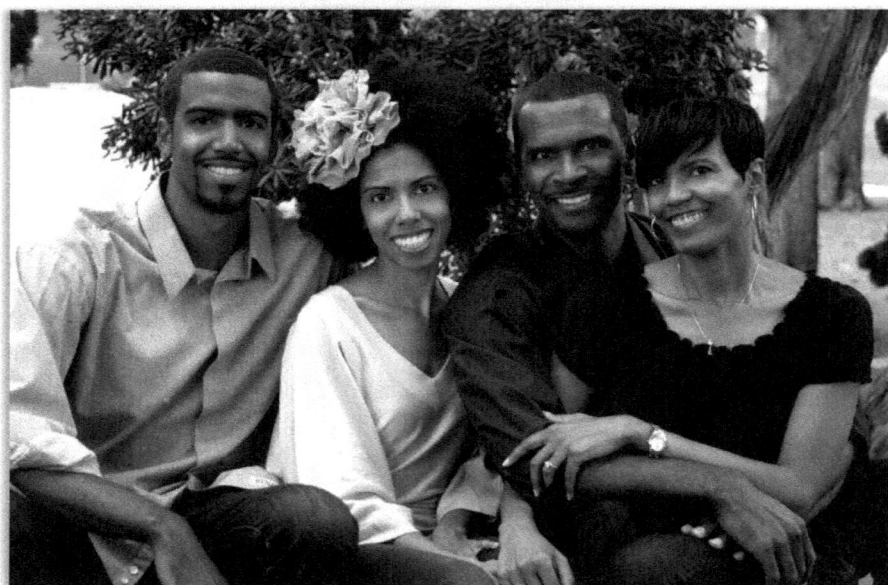

6

V

Quick and Easy Delicious Recipes!

These are some of my family's favorite recipes that are quick, delicious, and even a bit naughty (like the Fried Chick'n and the Vegan Carrot Cake!). We have a very balanced and flexible approach – all of our recipes are vegan but we do occasionnaly enjoy fried dishes and sweets, so I am including a couple of those recipes here. Remember that the most important thing is to adapt these recipes to your liking – make sure to play with the spices, add other ingredients, and even substitute sauces and condiments until you find the right balance for you. I can honestly say that I never use a recipe straight from a cookbook – I always play around with it until I know it will be perfect for my family's taste buds so you should do the same!

Check out the following dishes and see what intrigues you. Then get the products as listed in Chapter 5 – Vegetarian Shopping Guide, and go to work! You will have a vegan lunch or dinner on the table in no time!

For beautiful color photos of these amazing dishes download the
FREE eBook at
www.21stCenturyVegetarians.com.

Barbeque Seitan

Vegan Deep Dish Pizza

Tofurky® Veggie Wraps

Tempeh Tuna Wraps

Fried Chik'n

Penne Pasta with Vegan Italian Sausage

Chik'n Taco Soup with Enchiladas

Sauteed Tofu

Vegan Carrot Cake

Barbeque Seitan

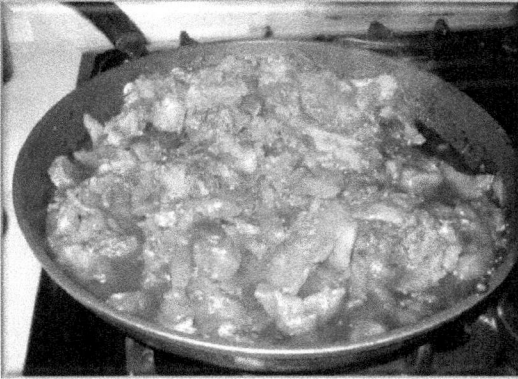

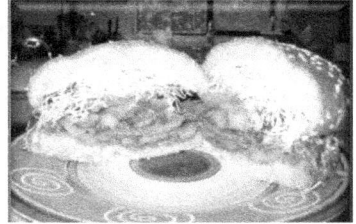

Seitan is made from wheat, is very high in protein, and has a surprisingly meaty texture. Try this recipe on a sandwich or a wrap!

INGREDIENTS

2 - 8oz packages of White Wave (Westsoy) Seitan (cubed or stir fry strips)

1/2 chopped sweet onion

About 2 cups of BBQ sauce of your choice. *(I use a combination of BBQ sauce, Soy Vay Teriyaki Sauce and Dragunara Sweet Chili Sauce - I like it sweet and spicy! However, any BBQ sauce will work).*

Small amount of Grapeseed oil for sautéing.

DIRECTIONS

Sauté the onions in a large pan or skillet until the onions are soft (about 2 min). Add the seitan, making sure that the liquid it is packed in is drained first. Add the BBQ sauce mix. Reduce the heat and let simmer about 5 - 7 min, stirring occasionally. Make sure the BBQ Sauce covers the seitan. You want to have enough sauce so that the seitan can soak it up.

After the seitan is tender and well marinated with the sauce, turn up the heat to "high" and quickly stir-fry the seitan. This will sear the sauce onto each piece and give it a more crispy texture and an authentic BBQ look.

That's it! You can put it on a sandwich (see photo above) or just have it as a side dish, with brown rice, on top of a salad, etc. The possibilities are endless!

Vegan Deep Dish Pizza

eBook Bonus

Watch the video! You Tube

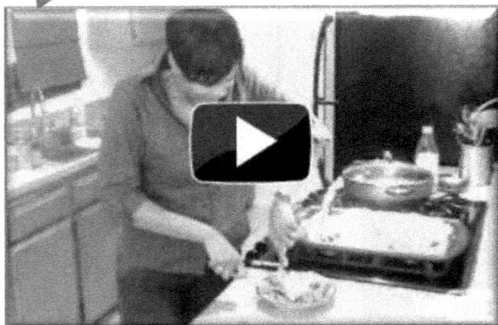

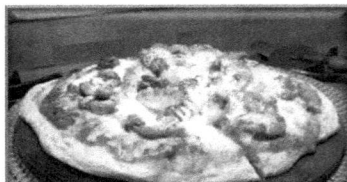

Pizza is one of my favorite foods yet I never found a deep dish vegan one that I really liked. Now, thanks to Daiya vegan cheese, my quest is over! We love this dish and hope that you do too!

INGREDIENTS

2 ready made pizza dough crusts - your choice of flavor
16 oz pizza or pasta sauce
4 cups vegan cheese * (I like Daiya Italian Blend)
½ cup chopped sweet onions
2 cups sliced mushrooms (I like crimini and portobello)
6 Tofurky® Italian Sausages - sliced
2 - 4 TBSP Italian Seasoning
2 cups chopped broccoli
1 cup chopped fresh pineapple (optional)
Oil for sautéing (I use grapeseed or canola)
You can use mozzarella cheese instead of the vegan cheese if you prefer a dairy option.

DIRECTIONS

Preheat oven to 450 degrees (or follow the directions on your pizza dough).

Remove the crusts from their wrapper and gently stretch the dough covering the bottom of a non-stick cookie sheet. Make sure that the dough is spread evenly so that there are no thin spots in the crust. Cover the crusts with a generous layer of pizza sauce. Cover the sauce with about half of the cheese, sprinkled evenly. Set aside.

In a large skillet, add a little oil (about 2 TBSP) and sauté the onions, mushrooms and Tofurky sausages for about a 1 - 2 minutes. Do not overcook. Add the Italian Seasoning (to taste) and the broccoli and sauté another minute or two. Do not overcook. You just want the sausages to be soft and juicy, and the broccoli lightly steamed.

When the vegetables are done, spoon them out on top of the pizza, ensuring even distribution. Add the pineapples if applicable. Cover with remaining cheese.

Place the pizza in the preheated oven for about 14 minutes, or according to the instructions on your pizza dough. NOTE: Each oven is slightly different - check on the pizza periodically to ensure that the cheese is not burning.

Remove the pizza and enjoy!

Serves 4 - 6.

Tofurky® Veggie Wraps

Watch the video! You Tube

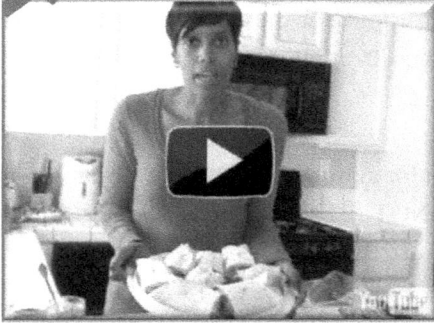

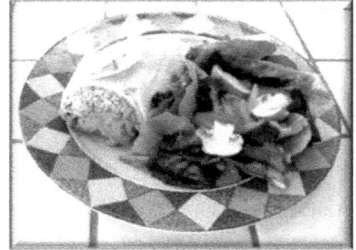

A fresh, delicious, easy and versatile recipe!

INGREDIENTS

1 package thinly sliced Tofurky® deli slices, Hickory Smoked flavor
3 large flour burrito wraps
Vegan Mayonnaise (I prefer Follow Your Heart Grapeseed Mayo)
1 TBSP. Mixed Grilled Vegetable Bruschetta (I use Trader Joe's or Whole Foods)*
1 TBSP. Corn and Chili Tomato-less salsa (I use Trader Joe's)*
½ small tomato, sliced
½ avocado, sliced
Miso Mayo, Spicy Red Pepper
1 large carrot (shredded)
Alfalfa Sprouts
Oil for sautéing (I use grapeseed or canola)
Optional

DIRECTIONS

Heat the tortillas and then set them aside. If you have a tortilla warmer that works fine. Otherwise, you can heat a little oil in a skillet and put each tortilla in the skillet for a few seconds until warm.

In the same skillet, add a little more oil (about 1 TBSP) and sauté the Tofurky slices for about a 1 - 2 minutes. Do not overcook. You just want them to become soft and juicy.

Spread a thin layer of the eggless mayonnaise on one wrap. Add about 5 slices of Tofurky in the middle of the tortilla, layering them so that you have a thin layer. Directly on top of the Tofurky, add the bruschetta, corn chili salsa, tomato and avocado.

Top with a thick squirt of the Miso Mayo, and then add the carrots and the sprouts. Fold each wrap at the ends, tuck in in the corners. Then fold the wrap lengthwise and gently squeeze it into a tight roll. Secure it with toothpicks and slice and enjoy!

Makes 3 wraps.

Tempeh Tuna Wraps

*This recipe was provided by my good friend and vegan chef, Marilyn Peterson from her book VEGAN BITE BY BITE (**www.veganbitebybite.com**). Kamaal and I spent some time cooking with Marilyn and learning how to prepare raw foods. This is one of her transition recipes and it's great! We love it because it's delicious, it's easy, and it's cheap!*

Note from Marilyn: *Tempeh is a fermented soy food high in protein, and easier to digest than tofu as it is less processed. It comes in a variety of different flavors, as well as "to go" burgers in the refrigerated section of natural food stores. The 'vegetable' flavor is great for this recipe. This is a great transitional recipe towards raw. This was a mainstay with me when I was transitioning to a higher percentage of raw foods in my diet.*

INGREDIENTS

1 8oz package tempeh, cut into 4 pieces (I like the Garden Veggie flavor)
1-1/2 cups celery, diced fine
1/2 cup green scallions, sliced fine
1/2 cup Vegenaise
1/4 cup lemon juice
2 tablespoons liquid aminos
1/4 teaspoon cayenne pepper
1 package whole wheat tortillas
Garnish: olives

DIRECTIONS

Pulse tempeh in food processor until fine. Put tempeh in a medium size bowl. Add the remaining ingredients, except tortillas and olives and mix together well.

Spread 1 teaspoon Vegenaise on each tortilla and layer 1 lettuce leaf with several sunflower sprouts. Spoon out less than 1/2 cup mixture evenly and spread it over the lettuce and roll the tortilla into a wrap. Garnish with an olive and serve.

Yield 2-1/2 cups or 6 wraps

Fried Chik'n

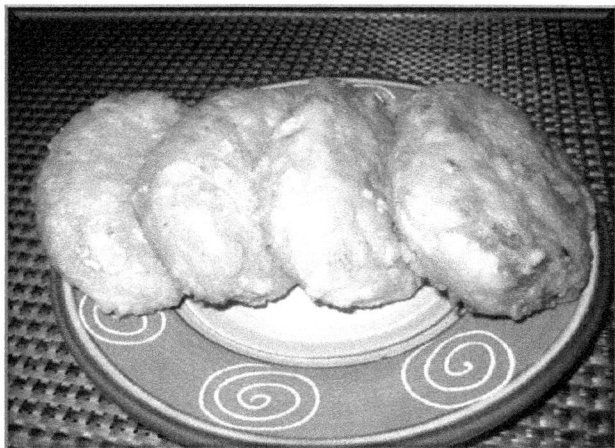

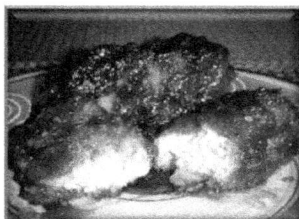

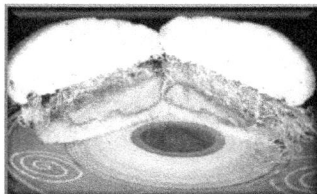

You know there had to be a vegan version of Fried Chik'n, right? That was very high on my conversion list! Hope you like it – try the BBQ version also or make a sandwich or wrap out of them! These stay moist and delicious for days.

INGREDIENTS

8 pcs Gardein Chik'n "breasts"
2 cups flour
1 teaspoon salt
½ teaspoon garlic powder
1 teaspoon pepper
1 teaspoon Spike® (optional)
½ cup warm water
4 tablespoons yellow mustard
2 cups Barbeque Sauce (if you are doing the BBQ version)
Oil for frying (I use Grapeseed or Canola)

DIRECTIONS

In a small mixing bowl, combine flour, salt, and garlic powder, pepper and Spike®. Mix thoroughly. In another small bowl, mix the mustard with the water. Add 2 tablespoons of the flour mixture to the mustard and water and stir until the lumps of flour are smooth and you have a batter about the consistency of pancake batter.

Heat the oil in a large skillet (or deep fryer) on high heat. There should be enough oil in the skillet to cover the bottom and be about ½ inch deep.

Dip each Gardein slice into the mustard batter, and then into the flour mixture, and then once again in the mustard batter making sure that each slice is well coated. Fry each slice on both sides in oil until golden brown (about 5 minutes each side). Remove from heat and let them drain on paper towels to remove excess oil.

Put the Barbeque sauce in a small bowl and dip each slice in the sauce until they are well coated. Put them in a broiler pan and broil each side under high heat until crispy.

Makes 8 pieces.

Penne Pasta with Vegan Italian Sausage

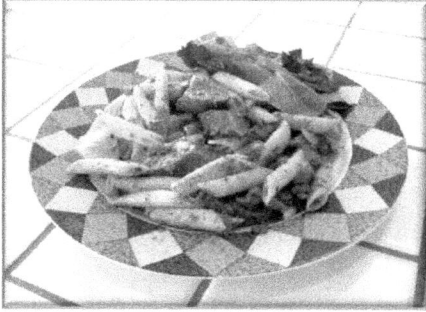

Very simple, delicious recipe that takes less than 30 minutes to cook. Full of protein and good carbs. Your family will love it!

INGREDIENTS

8 oz uncooked Penne Pasta
2 Tofurky® Italian Sausages
½ chopped onion
2 large Portobello Mushrooms, sliced (optional)
4 oz Sun Dried Tomatoes, julienne cut, packed in oil
8 oz Sun Dried Tomato Pesto or Tomato Bruschetta
1 teaspoon minced or crushed garlic (or ½ teaspoon garlic powder)
2 Tablespoons roasted red pepper pesto (optional)
2 Tablespoons Italian Seasoning (any brand should be fine)
Oil for cooking (I prefer Olive Oil for this recipe)

DIRECTIONS

Cook Penne Pasta according to package directions. Use a little oil in the water so the pasta won't stick. After cooking, rinse pasta and set aside.

Slice the Italian Sausage into bite sized pieces. In a large skillet, put a little cooking oil along with the oil from the sun dried tomatoes (drain the oil out of the jar of tomatoes). Heat oil mixture on high. Add the Italian Sausage, onion and mushrooms (if applicable). Add Italian Seasoning and garlic and sauté together for a few minutes until the onions are slightly brown and the Italian Sausage is crispy (about three minutes).

Add the sun dried tomatoes and continue cooking about one minute more. Add the cooked pasta to the mixture and stir to blend with the vegetables and the seasoning. Finally, add the sun-dried tomato pesto or (bruschetta) and the roasted red pepper pesto (if applicable) a little at a time. This pasta dish should be moist but not covered in pasta sauce so be careful not to add too much pesto. Cook for about one minute more and stir to blend the flavors and prevent sticking. Taste and add more Italian Seasoning if necessary.

Makes 2 - 3 servings. Goes great with Garlic Bread!

Chik'n Taco Soup with Enchiladas

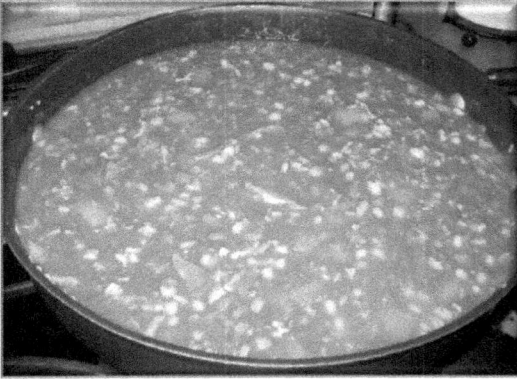

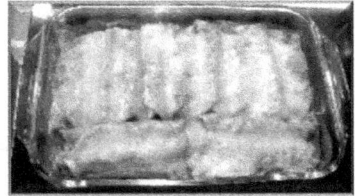

These are two VERY simple recipes that go great together and last for days! Makes great leftovers and is hearty and filling.

The soup recipe was given to me by my friend, Rod (thanks Rod!). Once I converted it to a vegetarian option, it became a family favorite!

INGREDIENTS FOR THE SOUP

1 chopped sweet onion

16oz Gardein® (chicken or steak style) – chopped fine in a food processor

1 package (1 ¼ oz) taco seasoning mix (I use ½ pkg mild and ½ pkg medium)

1 can (15 ½ oz) chili or baked beans

1 can (15 oz) tomato sauce

1 can (14 ½ oz) diced tomatoes – undrained

1 can (4.5 oz) chopped green chilis

1 package (1 oz) vegan ranch style dressing mix

1 16 oz package frozen sweet corn

4 cups water

Oil for frying (I use Grapeseed or Canola)

DIRECTIONS FOR THE SOUP

Sauté the onions in a large pan or skillet until the onions are soft (about 2 min). Add the Gardein and the taco seasoning mix. Continue cooking and stirring the mixture for about 2 – 3 minutes until the flavors blend.

Add the remaining ingredients, being sure to add the liquid from the beans and the tomatoes to the soup. Stir well and simmer, uncovered, over a low heat for about 15 minutes. That's it! You can eat this hearty soup by itself, over brown rice, or with enchiladas.

INGREDIENTS FOR THE ENCHILADAS

1 12 oz package Smart Ground® Veggie Crumbles – Mexican Style
1 dozen white corn tortillas
2 10 oz cans Red Enchilada Sauce (Medium Spiced)*
8 oz Daiya Vegan Cheese (cheddar blend)
9" x 13" baking dish
Earth Balance Buttery Spread

Enchilada sauce comes in mild and spicy also. Choose the flavor that suits you best.

DIRECTIONS FOR THE ENCHILADAS

Pre-heat oven to 375°. Put Smart Ground® Veggie Crumbles into a small bowl and set aside. In an iron or non-stick skillet, heat a small amount of the Earth Balance and lightly sauté one tortilla for a few seconds, flipping it once. This is just to moisten and soften it up.

Remove the tortilla from the pan and put one tablespoon of the Mexican Style Veggie Crumbles in the center of it, spreading it out so that it forms a line down the center. Put one tablespoon of Daiya cheese on top of the Veggie Crumbles, and roll the tortilla tightly, then place it in the baking dish. Repeat this process for the remaining tortillas.

When all tortillas have been placed into the baking dish, open each can of enchilada sauce and pour over the tortillas. The tortillas should be saturated. Sprinkle the remaining cheese on top.

Bake, uncovered for 15 minutes, or until cheese is thoroughly melted. Remove from oven and let cool. Garnish with guacamole and vegan sour cream if desired, or just eat as is. Makes one dozen enchiladas.

My family loves this dish because it tastes great. I love it because it is super simple! The Mexican Style of Smart Ground® is perfectly seasoned already and requires no preparation. What could be easier?

Quick and Easy Delicious Recipes! | 51

Sauteed Tofu

What would a vegetarian starter kit be without at least one tofu recipe? We actually love tofu but contrary to popular belief, this is not all we eat. Try this simple recipe but be sure to plan ahead – it requires that the tofu be frozen and thawed before cooking (see below).

THE "TRICK" TO TOFU

To get firm tofu that absorbs succulent flavors, try this simple trick!

1) Freeze the tofu overnight. Leave it in its original container.

2) Let the tofu thaw, still in its original container. For example, if you want to cook a tofu dish for dinner, take the frozen tofu out of the freezer in the morning and let it thaw, un-refrigerated, during the day. If you do not cook the tofu that evening, simply refrigerate it and it will stay fresh for several days.

3) After it thaws, remove the tofu from the plastic tub. You may decide to cook some now and some later. If you want to cook some later, put it in airtight Tupperware and add enough fresh water to cover the tofu. Re-refrigerate.

4) For tofu that you are ready to cook now, squeeze out the excess water. I like to do this by placing the block of tofu between two small plates and GENTLY pressing out as much of the water as possible. The tofu will take on a sponge-like consistency and is now ready to use in your favorite recipe!

INGREDIENTS

1 14oz container of extra firm tofu, frozen, thawed, and excess water squeezed out (per above instructions)
Spike® Seasoning (you can also use Salt Free Spike for lower sodium)
Bragg's Liquid Aminos® (Spray Bottle is most convenient)
Oil for Cooking (I prefer grapeseed)

DIRECTIONS

Make sure excess water is squeezed out of the tofu completely by placing the block of tofu between two plates and gently pushing them together. Be careful not to crush the tofu. Slice crosswise into pieces about ¼ inch thick.

Heat oil on high heat in a large iron skillet or frying pan. Use just enough oil to cover the bottom of the pan. Add tofu slices (if you have too many slices you may have to do this in two rounds). Spray Liquid Aminos over tofu slices so that they are lightly covered. Shake Spike over the tofu slices so that they are generously covered. Sauté tofu until it is crispy on the bottom, then flip each slice. Spray other side with Liquid Aminos and Spike and sauté until the other side is crispy. Flip once more just to blend the spices on each side.

Remove from skillet and place on paper towels to drain excess oil.

Makes 2 servings.

This is a great, high protein light meal that can be served for breakfast, lunch, or dinner. We like this in the evening with sautéed vegetables such as asparagus, broccoli, or brussel sprouts.

Vegan Carrot Cake

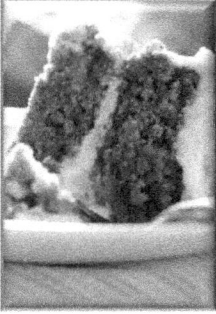

This is delicious, super-moist vegan carrot cake that has three elements; the cake, the glaze, and the frosting. It's super easy and absolutely a favorite of ours and our friends. It is actually VERY easy to make and worth the effort!

NOTE: to maximize time, make the glaze and the frosting while the cake is baking.

INGREDIENTS

CAKE
1 cup white sugar
½ cup brown sugar
1 ¼ cups vegetable oil
3 cups all-purpose flour
½ teaspoon salt
3 teaspoons baking powder
2 teaspoons baking soda
1 ½ teaspoons cinnamon
Dash of nutmeg
1 ½ cups soy or almond milk (vanilla)
2 teaspoons vanilla extract
2 cups raw grated carrot
1 cup chopped walnuts
1 cup raisins)

GLAZE
½ cup vegan creamer (I use Silk French Vanilla)
1 ½ tablespoons light corn syrup
1 ½ cups white sugar

FROSTING
4 oz Tofutti "Cream Cheese" – plain
¼ cup Earth Balance Whipped Buttery Spread
1 teaspoon finely grated lemon peel
2 ¼ cups powdered sugar

DIRECTIONS

For The Cake
Preheat the oven to 350°. Grease and flour a bundt or a 9 x 13 inch pan.

In a large bowl, mix the white sugar, brown sugar, and oil. Beat until light and fluffy. In another bowl, sift the flour, salt, baking powder, baking soda, cinnamon and nutmeg. Add the flour mixture to the sugar and oil and beat. Add the soy or almond milk and mix well.

Add the vanilla extract and stir again. Add the carrots and mix well. Finally, add the walnuts and raisin and mix all of the ingredients together until the batter is consistent.

Pour the batter into the pan and bake for about 45-55 minutes. Do not over bake! Check the cake after 45 minutes; if a toothpick is slightly moist after inserted into the middle of the cake, then it is ready. If necessary, bake another 10 minutes (a 9x13 pan will typically be done sooner than a bundt cake pan). When the cake is done, remove it from the oven and let it cool slightly (about 10 minutes), then add the glaze.

For The Glaze
Combine all of the glaze ingredients in a small bowl. Simply mix or stir until the ingredients are blended.

After the cake has cooled slightly, make a few holes in the top of the cake with a toothpick, and with a knife, gently separate the cake from the edges of the pan. Slowly pour the glaze on top of the cake and in the space between the cake and the edge of the pan. It should ooze all over the cake and seep in which will make it moist and even sweeter. Let the cake stand in the glaze for about an hour, and then gently remove the cake from the pan to finish cooling.

For The Frosting
In a saucepan or small pot, heat the Tofutti cream "cheese", Earth Balance "butter", and lemon peel over low heat until the butter is melted and the cream cheese is very soft.

In a medium bowl, add the powdered sugar. Add the cream cheese/butter mixture and blend or whisk together with the powdered sugar until the mixture is very smooth. Refrigerate the frosting for a few minutes until is it cooled and slightly stiff. Spread the frosting on the cake after it has cooled.

To my mind, the life of a lamb is no less precious than that of a human being. I should be unwilling to take the life of a lamb for the sake of the human body.

Mahatma Gandhi

Becoming Vegetarian

An Excerpt from
Orange Sunshine: How I Almost Survived America's Cultural Revolution,
by Marc DuQuette

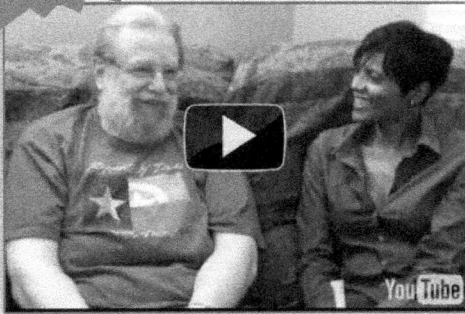

Marc is one of my dearest friends and has been a vegetarian for over 40 years. His memoir, Orange Sunshine: How I Almost Survived America's Cultural Revolution, *chronicles his journey during the 1960's and 70's, from self-destruction to self-discovery. It is an amazing book that is shocking yet hilarious!* Check out our interview where I ask Marc about *how he became a vegetarian,*

For more this and other interviews, book excerpts and reviews, visit Marc's site at **www.MarcDuQuette.com**, and see additional information at the end of this chapter.

A few weeks after my introduction to LSD, I attended a "love-in" held in a park in the San Fernando Valley.

I still had the biker mentality and affect, but I was becoming very curious about the hippie movement. It was late 1966, and there weren't many hippies in Orange County, so I began to hang out in Los Angeles on weekends.

I wandered around the park, staring at the hippies in their colorful outfits. Beads, bells, fringy leather shit, flowers in their hair – Really! I wasn't too out of place with my long hair and full beard, but the knife on my belt looked a little harsh.

A hippie girl, wearing a long tie-dyed dress handed me a pamphlet on vegetarianism. I glanced down at it and snapped at her, "Doesn't a carrot scream when you pull it out of the ground?" I had recently watched a scientific study on television, which seemed to prove plants could sense pain, danger and fear, as well as love and nurturing. I felt so smug, smarting-off to this gentle young woman. She just smiled in my direction and floated away.

The next weekend, my brother and I dropped some more acid. I don't remember why, but the trip turned into a bummer for me. Lon seemed to be doing O.K., but I was having trouble relating to planet Earth.
I thought maybe a hamburger and a beer would bring me back to the version of reality I was familiar with – "ground" me, in other words.
We jumped into my Chevy Malibu. I fired up the little 283 engine, fumbled with the four-on-the-floor shifter, and pointed us toward the nearest café that had a beer license.

I had difficulty driving on acid. On this particular trip, it seemed I had become the Incredible Shrinking Man, grasping my huge steering wheel. My brother appeared to be about ten feet away in the passenger seat. His head was enormous, and I could see every pore in his face. We must be aliens, I thought.

Somehow, we made it safely to the café, found a booth, and ordered our hamburgers and beer. When the nice lady from Earth in her crisp white uniform, brought the burgers, I took a big juicy bite out of mine.
I experienced the whole hamburger story – and more! My years in Nebraska – the gentle cattle with their big sad eyes. The pig I saw slaughtered alive by my alcoholic uncles near Julesburg, Colorado, when I was eight-year-old. I remembered it was an unbearably hot muggy day, out on the farm. The poor pig just wouldn't die. The horrible, pitiful sounds – it all came back – magnified and amplified.

I put my hamburger down and finished my Schlitz. I ordered two more bottles of beer, chugged them, and gave up eating meat and killing animals for food or sport. Vegetarianism became my "cause" for a few days, until I remembered my reaction to the hippie girl at the love-in. I had to laugh at myself.

ABOUT ORANGE SUNSHINE: HOW I ALMOST SURVIVED AMERICA'S CULTURAL REVOLUTION

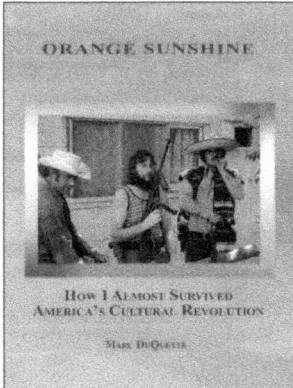

$19.99
Paperback, 204 pages
www.MarcDuquette.com

Get in, hold on, and shut up!

This wonderful baby-boomer-gone-wild autobiography captures the essence of 1960s America and beyond. I followed the karma of Marc DuQuette in one sitting, hanging on as he careened wildly from one adventure to the next, making me laugh and breaking my heart. It's worth the read simply to get inside the head of a man who will think to himself, upon being thrown to the ground by police, "What's the karma with my nose and the street?" I loved this book.

Melissa B. Latimer, Riverside, CA

A Veteran of the 1960's psychedelic revolution reveals the true story of the American Counterculture. How does a 22 year old alcoholic, drug-using outlaw biker/machine shop worker, in a span of less than three years, become a yoga practicing, vegetarian commune founding revolutionary, who, inspired by his psychedelic drug trips, begins to practice an Eastern form of meditation in search of inner peace? This sort of radical transformation could only take place during the 1960's Cultural Revolution, arguably America's most turbulent time when our country exploded into chaos and mad idealism. Orange Sunshine, How I Almost Survived America's Cultural Revolution, is the first hand account of what it was like to be an active participant in the movement that shaped our nation - a war baby's roller coaster ride of hot rods, guns, dope, revolution and redemption that's action-packed and heartbreakingly hilarious.

Born in 1942 in Long Beach, California, Marc's sense of patriotism and desire to be of help to his fellow man launches him on a spiritual quest, resulting in his hitting bottom - morally and spiritually. In Orange Sunshine, Marc writes with wit and honesty about his experiences, revealing a very personal, yet universally appealing, perspective on the chaos and turmoil of this country's most disaffected generation of the 20th Century. Today? Marc has been an addictions counselor for over twenty years. He lives in Southern California, and frequently travels to India to recharge his spiritual batteries.

I have no doubt that it is a part of the destiny of the human race, in its gradual improvement, to leave off eating animals, as surely as the savage tribes have left off eating each other.

Henry David Thoreau, Walden, 1854

Vegetarian Resources

The following is a list of incredible resources that my family and I highly recommend. We hope you will find them as helpful as we have!

WEBSITES

21st Century Vegetarians , *The Theus Family's Guide to Vegetarian Living*
www.21stcenturyvegetarians.com

ABC Health Food Markets, *Official site of the nonprofit online vegetarian store that offers a selection of vegetarian recipes, food, news, and more*
www.vegefood.com

Amy's Kitchen, *great vegetarian meals that have been a godsend to us!*
www.amyskitchen.com

Black Vegetarian Groups
> Black Vegetarians - www.blackvegetarians.org
> Black Vegetarian Society of Brooklyn -
> > http://groups.yahoo.com/group/blacksocietyofvegetarians/
> Black Vegetarian Society of Georgia - www.bvsga.org
> Black Vegetarian Society of New York - www.bvsny.org
> Black Vegetarian Society of North Carolina - www.myspace.com/bvsonc
> Black Vegetarian Society of Texas - www.bvstx.org/
> Houston Black Veggies -
> http://groups.yahoo.com/group/blackveggies/

By Any Greens Necessary , *from author Tracye Lynn McQuiter, MPH*
www.byanygreensnecessary.com

Compassion Over Killing
www.tryveg.com

European Vegetarian Union
www.euroveg.eu

Happy Cow Vegetarian Guide, *guide to health food stores and restaurants*
www.happycow.net

International Vegetarian Union, *information for vegetarians globally*
www.ivu.org

Meatless Monday, *from Johns Hopkins School of Public Health*
www.meatlessmonday.com

Organic Consumers Association
www.organicconsumers.org

People for the Ethical Treatment of Animals (PETA)
www.peta.org
www.goveg.com
www.peta.tv

Physicians Committee for Responsible Medicine
www.pcrm.org
Vegetarian Starter Kit - www.pcrm.org/health/veginfo/vsk/vsk.pdf
Vegetarian Diets for children -
www.pcrm.org/health/veginfo/veg_diets_for_children.html

Powered By Produce – *great blog!*
www.poweredbyproduce.com

Quarry Girl, *awesome site for vegan dining in Los Angeles*
www.quarrygirl.com

The Raw Mocha Angels, *Althea Hughes Wills blog which is packed with information about vegan soul food that is raw or gluten - free!*
www.therawmochaangel.blogspot.com

Symbiotic Wellness, *website of Valerie McGowan, Holisitic Health Counselor and Vegan, She's amazing and understands the benefits of a vegan diet!*
http://websites.integrativenutrition.com/vmcgowan/Home/Index.aspx

Sistah Vegan, *by author Breeze Harper. The Sistah Vegan Project focuses on how plant-based consumptive lifestyle is affected by factors of race, racisms, sexism, heterosexism, classism, and other social injustices within the lives of black females.*
www.sistahvegan.wordpress.com

Sister Vegetarian, *Sister Vegetarian is a blog of encouragement for sisters to take back our health.*
www.sistervegetarian.blogspot.com

Vegan Guinea Pig, *from author Alicia C. Simpson*
www.veganguineapig.blogspot.com

The Vegetarian Athlete, *also by author Martha Theus*
www.thevegetarianathlete.com

Vegetarians In Paradise, *excellent Los Angeles vegetarian guide*
www.vegparadise.com

Vegetarian Resource Group
www.vrg.org

The Vegetarian Site, *extensive online store offering vegetarian and vegan items*
www.thevegetariansite.com

The Vegetarian Society
www.vegsoc.org

Vegetarian Teen
www.vegetarianteen.com

Veggie Brothers
www.veggiebrothers.com

Veg News, *the popular vegan magazine*
www.vegnews.com

Viva Vegie Society, Inc.
www.VivaVegie.org
101 Reasons Why I'm a Vegetarian, by Pamela Rice - www.vivavegie.com/101.

BOOKS

Barnard, Dr. Neal, *Dr. Neal Barnard's Program For Reversing Diabetes*. New York, NY. Rodale Books, 2007.

Brazier, Brendan, *Thrive: The Vegan Nutrition Guide To Optimal Performance In Sports and Life*. Da Capo Lifelong Books, 2008.

Burroughs, Stanley, *The Master Cleanser*. Copyright 1976 and 1993, Stanely Burroughs and Alicia Burroughs, respectively.

Campbell, T. Colin and Campbell, Thomas M. II, *The China Study: Startling Implications For Diet, Weight Loss and Long-Term Health.* Dallas, TX. Benbella Books, 2006.

Davis, Gail, *So, Now What do I Eat?* (Copyright 1998 by Gail Davis).

Dorfman, Lisa, *The Vegetarian Sports Nutrition Guide: Peak Performance for Everyone from Beginners to Gold Medalists* (Copyright 1999).

DuQuette, Marc, *Orange Sunshine: How I Almost Survived America's Cultural Revolution.* Laguna Beach, CA. Copyright 2008, Marc DuQuette.

Foer, Jonathan Safran, *Eating Animals.* New York, NY. Little, Brown and Company, Hachette Book Group, 2009.

Freston, Kathy, *Quantum Wellness: A Practical and Spiritual Guide To Health and Happiness*. New York, NY. Weinstein Books, 2008.

Gerson, Charlotte and Walker, Morton, *The Gerson Therapy®: The Proven Nutritional Program For Cancer and Other Illnesses*. New York, NY. Kensington Books, 2001, 2006.

Gerson, Max, M.D. *A Cancer Therapy: Results of Fifty Cases & The Cure of Advanced Cancer by Diet Therapy, Sixth Edition.* San Diego, CA. The Gerson Institute, Copyright 1958, 1999, 2002.

Joy, Melanie, *Why We Love Dogs, Eat Pigs, and Wear Cows: An Introduction to Carnism, The Belief System That Enables Us To Eat Some Animals and Not Others.* San Francisco, CA. Conari Press, 2010.

Lappé, Anna and Terry, Bryant, *Grub: Ideas for an Urban Organic Kitchen* (Copyright 2006).

Lyman, Howard F., *No More Bull!* Voice for a Viable Future, 2005.

McQuirter, Tracye Lynn, MPH, *By Any Greens Necessary: A Revolutionary Guide For Black Women Who Want To Eat Great, Get Healthy, Lose Weight, and Look Phat.* Chicago, IL. Lawrence Hill Books, 2010.

Moskowitz, Isa Chandra, *Vegan With a Vengeance* (Copyright 2005).

Moskowitz, Isa Chandra and Romero, Terry Hope, *Vegan Cupcakes Take Over the World* (Copyright 2006).

Peterson, Marilyn, *Vegan Bite By Bite*, Los Angeles, CA. 3 Ton Tomato Press, 2010.

Rice, Pamela, *101 Reasons Why I'm a Vegetarian.* Viva Vegie Society, Eighth Edition, Copyright 2009. www.vivavegie.org/101.

Robbins, John, *Diet For A New America: How Your Food Choices Affect Your Health, Happiness, And The Future of Life on Earth.* (Copyright 1987 by John Robbins).

Robbins, John, *The Food Revolution: How Your Diet Can Help Save Your Life and Our World* (Copyright 2001).

Robbins, John, *Healthy at 100: How You Can – At Any Age – Dramatically Increase Your Life Span and Your Health Span.* New York, NY. Ballantine Books, 2006.

Simpson, Alicia C., *Quick and Easy Vegan Comfort Food.* New York, NY. The Experiment, 2009.

Singer, Peter and Mason, Jim, *The Ethics of What We Eat* (Copyright 2006 by Peter Singer and Jim Mason).

Terry, Bryant, *Vegan Soul Kitchen: Fresh, Healthy, And Creative African-American Cuisine*. Cambridge, MA. De Capo Press, 2009. (Copyright 2009 by Bryant Terry).

Wolfe, David, *Superfoods: The Food and Medicine of the Future.* Berkeley, CA. North Atlantic Books, 2009.

DVDs and MOVIES

Colquhoun, James and Laurentine ten Bosch, *Food Matters.* 2008.

Friedrich, Bruce, *Meet Your Meat*. 2003.

Greenstreet, Steven, *Killer at Large: Why Obesity is America's Greatest Threat,* 2008.

Kenner, Robert, *Food, Inc.* 2009 www.foodincmovie.com.

Koons, Deborah, *The Future of Food*. 2004.

Kroschel, Steve, *Dying to Have Known*. 2006.

Kroschel, Steve, *The Beautiful Truth*. 2008.

Monson, Shaun, *Earthlings.* Nation Earth, 2005. Narrated by Joaquin Phoenix. Music by Moby

Spurlock, Morgan. *Super Size Me*. Sony Pictures, 2004.

MORE INFORMATION ON THE WEB

A Global Stampede to the Meat Counter, Appleby, Paul.
www.ivu.org/oxveg/Publications/Oven/Articles_General/wi_meat.html

ADA (American Dietetic Association) Position Paper on Vegetarianism
www.vrg.org/nutrition/ada1993.htm

Ask The Vegan Athlete, an interview by Vegetarians in Paradise of Brendan Brazier, author of Thrive: The Vegan Nutrition Guide
www.vegparadise.com/athlete1.html

Body Building – Meatless Muscle, article by vegetarian body builder David Faircloth posted on the European Vegetarian Union website.
www.europeanvegetarian.org/evu/english/news/news002/meatless_muscle.html

Eat Better, Perform Better - Sports Nutrition Guidelines for the Vegetarian,
By Enette Larson, M.S., R.D. This article is presented by The Vegetarian Resource Group and has information about what to eat before, during, and after competition or training.
www.vrg.org/nutshell/athletes.htm

Fit Nation – Obesity Map (by CNN)
http://edition.cnn.com/SPECIALS/2007/fit.nation/obesity.map/

Growth and Development of Vegetarian Children, European Vegetarian Union
www.europeanvegetarian.org/evu/english/news/news972/children.html

Muscling Out the Meat Myth, by Dr. T. Colin Campbell, Phd, author of The China Study
www.vsdc.org/meatmyth.html

Protein in the Vegan Diet, an article by The Vegetarian Resource Group with information and charts about protein requirements of vegans.
www.vrg.org/nutrition/protein.htm

Rearing Cattle Produces More Greenhouse Gases Than Driving Cars, United Nation Report Warns, UN News Centre, November 29, 2006
http://www.un.org/apps/news/story.asp?NewsID=20772&Cr=global&Cr1=environment#

Veganism and the Issue of Protein, presented by P.E.T.A.
www.peta.org/issues/Animals-Used-for-Food/veganism-and-the-issue-of-protein.aspx?

Vegetarian Diets from the Viewpoint of Preventive Medicine and Dietics,
Dr.Mitsuru Kakimoto
www.ivu.org/news/march2000/diets.html

The Vegetarian Resource Group Nutrition Informaton - this is a great list of all sorts of vegetarian nutrition information such as iron in the vegetarian diet, gluten-free cuisine, and protein in the vegetarian diet.
www.vrg.org/nutrition/index.htm

Who Says You Have to Eat Meat to be a Successful Athlete? Sports Illustrated writer Jonah Keri's article featuring Tony Gonzalez, Prince Fielder, and other vegetarian/vegan athletes.
http://sports.espn.go.com/espn/page2/story?page=keri/080616

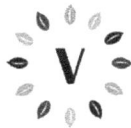

ABOUT MARTHA AND KAMAAL THEUS

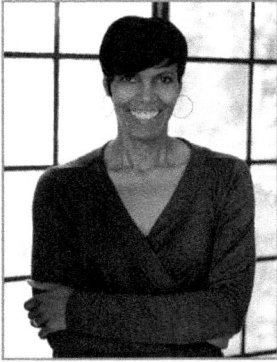

Martha Theus

I've been a vegetarian since 1985. I was raised in Detroit, Michigan, and introduced to a vegetarian way of life when I moved to Los Angeles and met my husband, Londale Theus, who has been a vegetarian since 1982.

Together, we raised our children, Kamaal and Londale Jr. as vegetarians since birth. Kamaal has graduated college and Londale is in his senior year. They are active, athletic, healthy young adults who have never eaten meat, poultry, fish or eggs, and I was fully vegetarian throughout both pregnancies.

As a young wife and mother, my goal was to create healthy and delicious food that does not involve pain and suffering for animals, yet tasted good and had a southern flair which reflects my roots. Over twenty years of trial and error, I feel that we have achieved this goal, and due to the request of so many of our family members and friends, my daughter Kamaal and I wrote Throwin' Down Vegetarian Style! in 2007 which is a collection of my favorite quick, easy, high protein vegetarian soul food and ethnic recipes. Since then, we have written two additional books and will release the second edition of Throwin' Down Vegetarian Style! in November 2010.

I believe Kamaal and I have "cracked the code" and taken the mystery and confusion out of vegetarian living by providing tips and recipes that are not only healthy but also very hearty and tasty and reminiscent of the foods we all grew up with.

My family and I are committed to a vegetarian lifestyle as a spiritual choice. I feel this lifestyle is a great blessing, as my family and I enjoy good health and we do not have any of the diet related diseases that many African Americans suffer from. We don't believe that you have to choose between eating "good" and eating "right." You can do both! You can find more information about us and how we live and eat at www.VeggieSoulFood.com or email me at Martha@VeggieSoulFood.com.

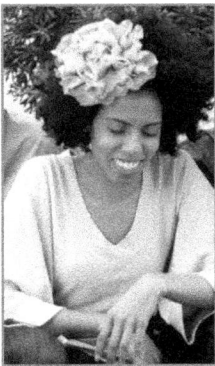

Kamaal Theus

Kamaal was born and raised is the suburbs of Los Angeles, and has been vegetarian since birth. She is an animal lover and has a passion for Japanese animation (anime), foreign cultures, and fashion. She is a recent graduate of California State University, Long Beach with a degree in Spanish Translation and Interpretation. She spent her freshman year in Costa Rica where she lived with a family, studied in the local university, and gained fluency in the language. Since that time, she has played college rugby, studied French and Japanese, visited Japan, and shared her vegetarian lifestyle with friends and co-workers from across the globe. Kamaal is the co-author of all of our books and is an integral part of the 21st Century Vegetarians business.

Photos by Brennen Scott, Brennen Scott Photography

www.ingramcontent.com/pod-product-compliance
Lightning Source LLC
Chambersburg PA
CBHW071837020426
42331CB00007B/1766